Notes on Medical Nursing

Notes on Medical Nursing

William C. Fream

M.B., B.S., S.R.N., B.T.A. Cert. (Hons), S.T.D., F.C.N.A.

General Practitioner,
Casterton, Victoria, Australia.
Formerly Senior Nurse Tutor,
Ballarat Base Hospital, Victoria, Australia.

THIRD EDITION

CHURCHILL LIVINGSTONE
EDINBURGH LONDON MELBOURNE AND NEW YORK 1982

CHURCHILL LIVINGSTONE
Medical Division of Longman Group Limited

Distributed in the United States of America by Churchill
Livingstone Inc., 19 West 44th Street, New York, N. Y.
10036, and by associated companies, branches and
representatives throughout the world.

First edition 1971
Second edition 1977
Third edition 1982

ISBN 0 443 02422 7

British Library Cataloguing in Publication Data
Fream, William C.
    Notes on medical nursing. — 3rd ed.
    — (Churchill Livingstone notes on nursing)
    1. Pathology
    I. Title
    616' 0024613   RT65

Library of Congress Catalog Card Number 81-82936

Printed in Singapore by Kyodo Shing Loong Printing Industries Pte Ltd

Preface to the Third Edition

Notes on Medical Nursing continues to be well received and many students have written to me to tell me what help they have gained from it. Many of their suggestions have been incorporated in this new edition. With their help the dilemma of what to include and what to omit has been reduced, although, with the welter of new information constantly arriving, the task is still hard.

Now that I am no longer actively engaged in nurse education I welcome most heartily any correspondence from those who are, especially if they feel they can help to improve my book in any way.

1982   W.C. Fream

Preface to the First Edition

The value to students of books in synoptic form has been realized in most professions for many years and it is surprising that the format has been used so little for nursing subjects. Often my own students have remarked on their need for something concise to which they can refer when they are in their final stages of training and have to revise a great deal of information in a short time. They complain that dictionaries and encyclopaedias give only restricted definitions and that standard texts give too much information for quick revision. It is in an attempt to fill the gap that this book has been written.

It is assumed that users of the book will have a sufficient working knowledge of anatomy and physiology to make inclusion of these subjects in the text unnecessary, since this would have added considerably to its length. Although primarily intended for the senior student nurse, it is hoped that qualified nurses and paramedical staff, even those who have specialised, will also find the book useful for reference.

I would like to take this opportunity to thank Miss Margaret Bennett, Staff Tutor, College of Nursing, Australia, and Miss Nancy Roper for their inestimable help with the manuscript.

1971   W. C. Fream

Contents

1. The Cardiovascular System

Electrocardiogram (ECG)

An ECG is a graph of minute electric currents generated as electrolytes surge in and out of cardiac muscle cells during contraction. The curves are labelled P, Q, R, S and T waves. The P wave occurs when the SA node emits an impulse; the Q, R, S waves occur as the impulse spreads through the ventricles; the T wave occurs at end of refractory period. The whole pattern is called 'a complex' and represents changes occurring during one heart beat. Normally complexes occur at regular intervals. Variations from normal pattern occur in many heart diseases.

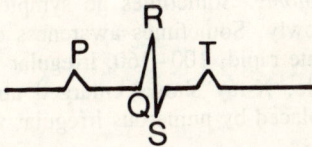

Distance between P and Q reflects length of time impulse takes to traverse conducting fibres between atria and ventricles. Normally distance less than 5 small squares (0·2 seconds). Increased in partial heart block, myocarditis, digitalis poisoning. Decreased in Wolff-Parkinson-White Syndrome.

QRS complex normally 3 small squares wide (0·12 seconds). Widening indicates prolongation in spreading of impulse, e.g. in myocarditis, ventricular hypertrophy.

Q waves normally small or missing. Large Q waves often present in myocardial infarction.

All waves are deviations from a basic line – iso-electric line. Elevation of this line between S and T occurs in myocardial damage.

T wave usually directed upwards from iso-electric line. Inverted T wave indicates myocardial ischaemia or old infarct.

Recording an ECG

Explain to patient what is about to happen stressing harmlessness of procedure and its freedom from any sensation. Patient should be at rest in warm environment. Skin should be free from contaminants, dressings, discharge. Leads placed in correct sequence firmly fixed with sufficient electrolyte paste or gel between electrode and skin. The chest leads should be positioned accurately keeping to exactly same routine with every recording. Strip kept under observation during recording and adjusted to keep graph central. Afterwards, wipe away electrode gel.

Conditions affecting the cardiac conducting mechanism

Atrial fibrillation

A condition in which impulses originate from many points in atrial myocardium instead of at SA node only.

Causes. Mitral stenosis; coronary insufficiency; hypertension; chronic nephritis; thyrotoxicosis; poisoning by bacterial toxins.

Signs and symptoms. Sometimes no symptoms especially if ventricles beat slowly. Sometimes awareness of irregular rate. Usually – pulse rate rapid, 100–160, irregular rate and rhythm. Apex beat forcible. X-ray shows enlarged atria. ECG shows absent P wave replaced by numerous irregular waves.

Diagnosis. ECG.

Types. *Paroxysmal*. Lasting hours to 2–3 days.

Established. Permanent unless treated with quinidine or procaine amide. If due to thyrotoxicosis – stops after correction.

Treatment. Digitalis to slow ventricular rate and strengthen ventricular force. Has no effect on atria which continue to fibrillate. Quinidine lengthens refractory period of atrial muscle cells and *may* stop fibrillation in selected cases. Procaine amide acts similarly but may cause fall in blood pressure. Procaine amide sometimes used prophylactically before operations when patient has a cardiac condition and the possibility of fibrillation is feared.

Cardioversion by d.c. countershock often used in new cases of atrial fibrillation [AF], when AF persists in patients whose thryotoxicosis has been controlled, when AF precipitates cardiac failure, or whenever it is thought patient's condition would be improved by sinus rhythm.

Shock administered to chest wall with patient anaesthetized 2·5 m sec, 10 to 400 watt-seconds, under cardiac monitor control. Shock causes systolic contraction of entire myocardium. Sinus node recovers from refractory period most rapidly and fires off next beat.

Prognosis. Always a serious condition putting a strain on ventricles. Atria are in a constant state of diastole hence great tendency for thrombi to form. Thrombi in right side of heart cause pulmonary emboli. From left side emboli may enter arteries and lodge in any part of body. Congestive cardiac failure a frequent termination.

Atrial flutter

A condition similar to fibrillation but atria contract regularly though incompletely. Atrial rate over 250 whereas in fibrillation it may be over 400. ECG in flutter shows regular pattern of P waves often with sawtooth appearance. Ventricular rate depends on whether impulses arriving at AV node do so during or after its refractory period. Pulse shows missed beats in regular order, sometimes every third beat. Causes may be similar to fibrillation but frequently idiopathic. Treatment by digitalis or quinidine may restore normal rhythm. Newer drugs used disopyramide (Rythmadon. Norpace).

Cardioversion may be used as in fibrillation.

Beta blockade commonly used to slow ventricular rate provided congestive cardiac failure absent.

Paroxysmal Supraventricular tachycardia

Sudden onset and cessation of regular tachycardia of 140–180 beats per minute due to either an ectopic atrial focus or to reactivation of normal pacemaker node by impulse returning through aberrant conduction pathway.

Occurs in otherwise healthy people. Often no discernible precipitating factor. Occasionally set off by excessive smoking, coffee, alcohol. Usually short duration but occasionally prolonged.

Patient often knows how to stop attack by stimulating vagal activity e.g. by carotid sinus pressure or irritating pharynx. If these measures unsuccessful digitalis, verapamil, or cardioversion may be tried. Verapamil (Isoptin) 5 mg i.v. given slowly usually stops attack immediately. Prevention of further attacks by beta blockers, verapamil or digitalis and avoidance of precipitating factors where these exist.

Heart block

Interruption of bundle of His or one of its branches so that impulses are delayed or fail to pass onwards.

Causes. Rheumatic fever. Diphtheria. Coronary occlusion. Digitalis toxicity. Endocarditis.

Grades of block. 1. Incomplete or partial. PR interval on ECG prolonged greater than 0·2 seconds.

2. Second degree heart block. Some atrial impulses get through conducting fibres, some do not. Usually block occurs regularly so that ventricles fail to contract at every third or fourth atrial contraction. (2:1 or 3:1 block).

3. Third degree or complete heart block. Atria and ventricles dissociated completely. ECG shows P waves occurring at regular intervals and QRS complexes occurring at slower rate independently of P waves.

Signs and symptoms. Depends on grade. Partial — may be discovered only with ECG.

Second degree. Usually regularly dropped ventricular beats with consequent pulse deficit.

Complete block. Ventricular rate about 40 to 50 per minute. Fainting attacks. Congestive cardiac failure.

Bundle Branch Block (BBB)

Bundle of His divides into two main branches, right to right ventricle and left which subdivides into antero-lateral and postero-inferior sub-branches to left ventricle.

Block of right bundle often found on ECGs of normal people. Left BBB indicated slow progress of impulse through myocardial fibres rather than rapid progress via conducting fibres.

Treatment. Drug treatment of heart block disappointing. Implantation of ventricular pacemaker.

Pacemakers

Pulse generator delivers impulse to ventricles. Generator may be external or implanted. External pacemaker often used for temporary pacing, e.g. in acute heart block, while implanted ones more suitable for permanent pacing.

Wire to ventricle may be passed internally to right ventricle via subclavian vein or can be embedded externally into ventricle.

Two common types of pacemaker are 'fixed rate' and 'demand'.

Fixed rate ones deliver impulses at a predetermined rate while demand pacemakers send out an impulse only when feedback from the ventricle indicates delayed intrinsic activity of myocardium.

Stokes–Adams syndrome

Occurs in patients with previous partial block when block suddenly becomes complete. Ventricles stop for several seconds until they start independently of atria. No pulse during cessation. Pallor, fainting, later cyanosis. Rapid recovery (if at all) with marked bradycardia. Treated with a pacemaker.

Cardiac arrest

Once considered irremedial. Now, in selected cases, if circulation maintained by cardiac massage and oxygenation maintained, ventricles may start beating again. Resuscitation should be started within 3 minutes of cardiac arrest otherwise irreversible changes take place in brain due to anoxia.

Place patient on firm surface — floor, fracture boards. Inferior part of sternum depressed forcibly 2–3 inches 60 times a minute. Mouth to nose breathing pending arrival of oxygen, mask and rebreathing bag. Mouth to nose breathing (with patient's mouth held closed) helps to keep tongue from blocking pharynx more readily than in mouth to mouth breathing.

Ventricular arrhythmias

Ventricular extra systole. Common phenomenon. Extra ventricular contraction occurs without prior atrial contraction. Next normal atrial impulse arrives at AV node during its refractory period and fails to penetrate. Hence there is a 'dropped beat' before normal rhythm resumed.

Incidence increases with intake of alcohol, smoking, coffee, strong tea, advancing age. Considered pathological if frequent. Danger sign in coronary insufficiency, myocardial hypertrophy, infarction. May proceed to lethal arrhythmia when occurring in conjunction with cardiac disease, or in association with overdosage of digitalis, quinidine, tricyclic antidepressants, or hypokalaemia.

Treatment. Remove cause. Cardioversion if frequent or in association with myocardial infarction — lidocaine (Xylocaine). 50 to 100 mg i.v. followed by 1 to 4 mg/minute i.v. infusion.

Beta receptor blockade i.v. dose depending on type of blocker used.

Other drugs sometimes used — procaineamide, quinidine, disopyramide, mexiletine.

Ventricular fibrillation is common cause of death in acute myocardial ischaemia.

Treatment is cardioversion. If there is likelihood of delay before patient can reach coronary care unit, injection of lignocaine 300 mg i.m. may help.

Long-term treatment with beta-blockers or sulfinpyrazone reduces incidence of sudden death in patients at risk.

Temporary pacing may be successful when drugs are not.

Drugs used in conditions affecting the conducting mechanism

Digitalis

Derived from foxglove plant (*Digitalis purpurea*).

Action. Lengthens refractory period of AV node. Slows ventricular rate. Strengthens ventricular force. Increases stroke volume. Whole circulation improves with benefit to oedema, urinary output, appetite, absorption, mental faculties. Does not change fibrillation.

Preparations. Tincture 0·6 ml. Powdered leaf 60 mg. Nativelles granules 0·1 mg. Digoxin — purified glucoside — most commonly used. Given i.v. for quick action 1 mg immediately then orally 0·25 mg 3 times daily reducing to 0·25 mg daily.

Overdosage. Pulse below 60. Beats may occur in pairs. Urine output diminished. Nausea and vomiting. Headache.

Treatment. Stop dosage until pulse about 70. Recommence with lower dose.

Quinidine

Related to quinine.

Action. Lengthens refractory period of cardiac muscle cells. Slows conduction of impulses by muscle cells. (If second action too marked it outweighs advantage of first and fibrillation continues. This is most likely to occur in enlarged hearts).

Contra-indications. Idiosyncrasy. Trial dose of 200 mg. If no nausea, sweating, headache, diarrhoea or rash, continue with full dosage. Unsuitable if there has been no improvement with digitalis; if fibrillation has existed for 6 months or longer; if heart is greatly enlarged. Previous symptoms of embolism indicate very real danger because sudden resumption of atrial systole may provoke serious embolism.

Dosage. 300 mg immediately, repeated once or twice at 2 hourly intervals. Second and third days 600 mg in 3 doses each day. Discontinue if regularity not restored. If regularity restored 300 mg daily for 2 to 3 weeks.

Procaine amide

Similar in action to quinidine but less danger of idiosyncrasy. Strengthens force of ventricles. Danger of sudden fall in blood pressure. May cause agranulocytosis. Oral tablets ½ – 1 g every 4 hours. Can be given i.v. or i.m.

Lidocaine (Xylocaine)

Stabilises myocardium when given i.v. 1 mg/kg in single dose followed by 1 to 4 mg/minute.

Beta adrenergic receptor blockers

Several slightly different chemical structures available — propranolol, pindolol, oxprenolol, alprenolol, etc. Slows heart rate and lengthens diastole hence myocardium receives longer period of nourishment via coronary circulation. Lowers blood pressure by relaxing arterioles and reducing peripheral resistance. Lowers cardiac output, therefore contraindicated in congestive cardiac failure. Causes bronchospasm hence contraindicated in asthma and chronic airways obstruction, though claims made for some newer β blockers that they are cardio-selective, i.e. they act on beta adrenergic receptors in heart more than on those elsewhere and may be safe to use in asthmatics — atenolol (Tenormin). Metoprolol (Betaloc. Lopressor).

Verapamil (Isoptin)

Calcium antagonist impedes transport of calcium ions across cell membranes. Extends refractory period thus slowing heart rate. Useful in tachycardias. Contraindicated in heart block, myocardial insufficiency, recent myocardial infarction. Not to be used with beta blockers.

May precipitate heart block, asystolic arrest, ventricular fibrillation and should not be given i.v. unless facilities available for resuscitation.

Dosage i.v. 5 mg slowly with constant observation of heart rate and blood pressure.

Oral 40–120 mg t.i.d.

Disopyramide (Norpace. Rythmadon)

Increases length of atrial refractory period and slows conduction through accessory pathways. Side effects due to anticholinergic properties are glaucoma, urinary retention, dry mouth, constipation, gassy distension.

Used to maintain normal rhythm after electro conversion and to prevent atrial tachycardia.

Dosage i.v. up to 150 mg over 10–15 minutes followed by infusion of up to 25 mg per hour in 5 per cent Dextrose.

Oral. Loading dose 200 to 300 mg then 100–150 mg 6 hourly.

Mexiletene

Similar to lignocaine but with advantage of oral administration.

Dosage. Oral 100–200 mg. t.i.d.

Can be given i.v. 250 mg statim and then by infusion 30–60 mg per hour but no advantage over lignocaine. May cause nausea, rashes and tremor.

Pericardium

Inflammatory heart disease: pericarditis

Inflammation of double sac of pericardium.

Causes. 1. Sterile inflammation from acute rheumatism, myocardial infarction, carcinoma, uraemia.

2. Infective. Streptococci, staphylococci, pneumococci, viruses. May be blood borne or contiguous from lungs and pleura.

3. Chronic inflammation. Almost always tubercular.

Stages. 1. Fibrinous exudation. Opposing surfaces shaggy with fibrin. Slippery surface destroyed. May last hours or days.

2. Serous exudation. Variable quantity of serous fluid poured into sac. May be clear and sterile or cloudy and purulent.

Signs and symptoms. Precordial pain. Creaking rub on auscultation. If fluid develops quickly and in large amount parietal pericardium does not have time to stretch and accommodate it. Pressure exerted on heart and prevents proper filling during diastole. Result is tachycardia, increased venous pressure — swollen neck veins, oedema, hepatic engorgement, portal back pressure, interference with digestion and absorption.

If fluid develops slowly sac dilates to accommodate it; venous congestion does not occur but enlarged heart displaces lung tissue causing dyspnoea, orthopnoea, cyanosis.

General symptoms if purulent — rigors, intermittent temperature, malaise.

Treatment. Rest. Treat underlying cause. Penicillin if purulent. Morphia during painful phase. Aspiration if amount large or if heart embarrassed.

Prognosis. Good with prompt treatment when purulent. Poor if accompanying myocarditis severe.

Constrictive pericarditis

Adhesions form between layers thus restricting movement. Overcome by hypertrophy of myocardium. Occasionally — great thickening of parietal layer with deposition of lime salts so that heart enclosed in rigid stony case. Mostly due to tuberculosis.

Other rarer causes — fungal and parasitic infections, radiation, rheumatoid arthritis, neoplastic disease.

Signs and symptoms. Venous obstruction — hepatic engorgement, portal obstruction, digestive disturbance, oedema, ascites, jugular pulsation, pounding headache.

Treatment. Removal of parietal pericardium especially round ventricles.

Acute myocarditis

Inflammation of myocardium.

Causes. 1. Acute toxaemia during course of diphtheria, scarlet fever, influenza, streptococcal infections, some viruses notably Coxsackie B or echoviruses.

2. Allergic response after streptococcal sensitization in acute rheumatism, chorea or acute nephritis.

Signs and symptoms. Low blood pressure. Pulse rapid and remains so while asleep. Sometimes atrial fibrillation. Malaise and weakness. May be asymptomatic and overshadowed by underlying disease.

Treatment. Absolute rest for 3–6 weeks. Treat underlying cause.

Cardiomyopathy

Disorder of myocardium of unknown cause.

Classification. 1. Congestive. Myocardium is thinned, dilated, contracts poorly.

2. Hypertrophic. Myocardium is thick, obstructing outward flow of blood. Contraction during systole is poor.

3. Restrictive. Myocardium is stiff due to fibrotic replacement of muscle cells or infiltration causing defective filling and poor systolic contraction.

Signs and symptoms. Cough, breathlessness, oedema, weakness.

Atrial fibrillation common.

Angina pectoris common in hypertrophic variety.

Treatment is that of failure — diuretics, peripheral vasodilator, e.g. hydralizine, isosorbide dinitrate, prazocin, salbutamol. Beta blockade is used for angina pectoris.

Endocarditis

Inflammation of the endocardium.

1. Acute bacterial endocarditis. Serious manifestation of septicaemia. Organisms from elsewhere — infected wound, whitlow, osteomyelitis, drug addiction — carried in blood stream and lodge in heart valves. Organisms commonly streptococci, staphylococci, pneumococci. Soft vegetations in valves may break off causing pyaemia and multiple abscesses anywhere.

Signs and symptoms. (Often masked by original infection). High fever; rigors; tachycardia; extreme toxaemia; delirium. When pyaemia occurs, toxaemia worse; localizing symptoms depending on site of lodgement of emboli; abscess formation.

Diagnosis. Blood culture.

Treatment. Mixed antibiotic therapy — penicillin, streptomycin, until sensitivity established, then massive doses of antibiotic to which organism sensitive.

2. Subacute bacterial endocarditis. Endocarditis occurring in people with an already damaged heart, e.g. following rheumatic fever or congenital lesions.

Cause. Almost invariably *Streptococcus viridans*. Occasionally *Strep. faecalis*, *Staph. pyogenes*, *Staph. aureus*, *Staph. albus*.

Occurrence. Following tooth extraction or tonsillectomy.

Signs and symptoms. Insidious onset with lassitude, anorexia, weight loss, anaemia. Embolism due to breaking off of soft vegetations from margins of affected valves. Smallest emboli may lodge in glomeruli causing haematuria, or in skin vessels causing petechiae which are important diagnostically. Brain — hemiplegia; kidney — infarct and anuria; limb — gangrene. Blood vessels may be weakened — aneurysms may occur. Low evening temperature; heart murmur; pallor; finger clubbing; enlarged spleen; Osler's nodes — painful red patches on finger pads; anaemia with leucocytosis. Splinter haemorrhages — linear haemorrhages under finger and toe nails.

Treatment. Prophylaxis important in people known to have had rheumatic fever or congenital heart lesions. Bicillin, ampicillin, gentamycin given i.v. or i.m. half-an-hour before procedure and 8 and 16 hours after. Curative — penicillin and streptomycin for 6 weeks. Observe carefully for 2–3 months to detect relapse early. Causative organism grown from blood culture. Antibiotic according to sensitivity.

Complications. Valvular incompetence. Congestive cardiac failure. Rupture of chordae tendinae. Perforation of valve cusps.

Rheumatic heart disease

In some people streptococcal infection may lead to sensitization of certain cells. Investigation now proceeding suggests that fibrous tissues are susceptible to development of 'auto-immunity' in which antibodies react abnormally with sensitized cells. Fibrous tissue occurs extensively in heart, hence high incidence of valvular disease following streptococcal infections. Acute rheumatism is another manifestation. Chorea is third.

Occasionally valvular incompetence arises acutely during rheumatic fever. Sudden back pressure into a normal left atrium is immediately transmitted to lungs causing acute pulmonary oedema.

Original attack of rheumatic fever may pass undiagnosed.

Valvular changes may then progress slowly over 10–15 years and patient is apparently well to 20–30 years of age.

Valvular heart disease: Mitral incompetence

Mitral valve becomes stiffened, thickened and inflamed. Coarse, warty vegetations develop and may cause emboli. Affected valve allows regurgitation, systolic murmur heard.

Mitral stenosis

Narrowing of mitral valve (buttonhole valve); left atrial dilatation. Presystolic murmur caused by turbulent flow through narrow opening as left atrium contracts. Back pressure along pulmonary veins causes engorgement of lungs, pulmonary oedema, cardiac asthma, dyspnoea, haemoptysis, thrombosis of pulmonary vessels and pulmonary infarct. (Left sided heart failure).

If untreated, backpressure throughout pulmonary circulation affects right side of heart and impedes progress of oncoming blood throughout venous system resulting in congestive cardiac failure.

Treatment. Curative treatment by valvotomy in suitable cases. Recently prosthetic valve replacements have proved effective. If surgery not possible — symptomatic treatment only. Easy life without additional strain on heart essential.

Complications. Bronchitis, emphysema, atrial fibrillation, embolism.

Aortic valve incompetence

Following inflammation valve pockets shrink and allow regurgitation from aorta to left ventricle during diastole. To maintain adequate circulation left ventricle hypertrophies enormously.

Causes. Rheumatic inflammation; syphilis; subacute bacterial endocarditis; dissecting aneurysm; ankylosing spondylitis.

Signs and symptoms. Before dilatation and hypertrophy of left ventricle — faintness on rising or stooping; poor memory; irritability due to cerebral anaemia. When hypertrophy established may be no symptoms. Signs show enlarged heart; apex beat forcible and often in 6th or 7th interspace instead of 5th; high systolic blood pressure; diastolic murmur; 'collapsing' pulse in which forcible thrust felt during systole falls away rapidly during diastole; visible capillary pulsation in nailbeds and lips.

Incompetence usually slowly progressive. Failure of ventricle eventually, though may take many years. When failure occurs — shortness of breath, cardiac pain similar to angina, cough, oedema of dependent parts.

Treatment. Encouraging results from replacement with prosthetic valves. Otherwise symptomatic treatment when failure occurs.

Aortic stenosis

Definition. Narrowing of outflow from left ventricle.

Incidence. Male:female ratio 4:1.

Causes. Anteriosclerosis. Rheumatic fever.

Signs and symptoms. In early stages left ventricular hypertrophy compensates for increasing obstruction and condition produces no symptoms or signs at this stage — ejection systolic murmur transmitted to neck and apex. Palpable thrill over right 3rd intercostal space.

Later when stenosis no longer overcome satisfactorily by increasing pressure exerted by left ventricle, cerebral insufficiency, angina, exertional dyspnoea, noticeable pounding sensation. Pulse pressure rises slowly to a low, soft amplitude.

ECG shows large R and S waves denoting ventricular hypertrophy. Large heart seen on X-ray. Often calcification present at aortic valve. Frequently aorta dilated and uncoiled.

Treatment. Prosthetic valve replacement in suitable case. In others, digitalis contraindicated as myocardium already contracting forcibly. Beta adrenergic receptor blockers slow rate allowing more time for perfusion of myocardium and reduce end-diastolic pressure within left ventricle.

Excision of portion of hypertrophied muscle improves cardiac performance if stenosis relieved surgically.

Other valvular lesions

Tricuspid valve. Rarely affected by rheumatic fever. When it is, usually combined with mitral disease. Undergoes similar progression. Stenosis, dilation of R. atrium, hypertrophy of R. ventricle.

Venous back pressure causes systemic symptoms, hepatomegaly, ascites, gross oedema, raised JVP.

Treatment. Valvotomy. Valve replacement. Diversion of blood from inferior vena cava to pulmonary artery.

Pulmonary valve. Almost never affected by rheumatic disease.

Pulmonary heart disease (cor pulmonale)

Anything impeding free flow of blood through pulmonary circulation causes strain on right ventricle which dilates and hypertrophies to overcome obstruction.

Causes. Breakdown of normal lung tissue, replacement with fibrous tissue — tuberculosis, pneumoconiosis, asbestosis, anthracosis. Breakdown of intra-alveolar septa and destruction of capillary bed — emphysema, cystic disease.

Signs and symptoms. Dyspnoea, especially on exertion, due to lack of respiratory surface; cyanosis; respiratory infections easily contracted; bronchitis; enlarged heart — right ventricular hypertrophy. As disease progresses — congestive cardiac failure, orthopnoea.

Treatment. Symptomatic. Avoid exertion. Treat infections promptly. Stop smoking.

Conditions preventing free flow of blood through coronary arteries: Atheroma

Deposits of fatty material form between tunica intima and tunica media. Tunica intima becomes soft and bulges into blood vessel lumen partially occluding it. Plaques of atheroma undergo fibrosis; lime is deposited in them. The result is atherosclerosis.

Thrombosis

The plaques bulging into the lumen cause back eddies in blood flow encouraging formation of thrombi. Sometimes a patch of atheroma erodes through tunica intima and destroys surface cells of squamous epithelium; blood clots on this rough surface.

Embolism

An embolus is any foreign substance floating in the blood. Emboli commonly responsible for occluding coronary vessels are associated with atheroma. Atheromatous plaques, having broken through the tunica intima, may then become dislodged and flow onwards to a place where the vessel becomes narrow. Such an embolus blocks the lumen and all that section of myocardium previously dependent on that particular vessel for its blood supply starves and dies. Other emboli may be derived from — warty vegetations on edges of mitral valve in rheumatic endocarditis; thrombi forming on the atrial walls during fibrillation; breaking down of myocardium following myocardial infarction.

Results of deficient blood flow through coronary arteries: Angina pectoris

Signs and symptoms. Pain unmistakable. Always comes on during exercise or raised emotional tone. Duration seconds to minutes, rarely more than 3 minutes. Distribution — typically retrosternal, radiating down inner border of left arm; occasionally up into neck and jaw; occasionally into right side of chest; occasionally into epigastrium. Described as 'crushing' pain 'as if heart is being squeezed'. Less and less exercise needed to initiate an attack. Occasionally sweating, vomiting.

Cause. Reduction in blood flow through coronary vessels, more especially those supply left ventricle, so that metabolic demand is not met. Blood flow satisfactory until extra demands made by exercise or emotional states. Most common cause — mechanical obstruction of coronary vessels by atheroma. Others: Severe aortic stenosis, hyperthyroidism, severe anaemia, increased viscosity as in polycythaemia, low blood pressure, greater myocardial bulk as in hypertrophy.

Treatment. During attack — rest lying down with one small pillow. Keep warm. Vasodilator drugs; amyl nitrite 3–5 minims, vapour inhaled; nitroglycerine (Trinitrin) tablets chewed slowly, retained in mouth for absorption from oral mucosa.

Possible in selected cases to improve blood flow to myocardium surgically, by bypassing stenosis of coronary vessel with venous or prosthetic graft.

Other causes corrected — anaemia, thyrotoxicosis, maintain adequate blood pressure.

Prevention of attacks. Lead quiet life free from domestic strife or business worries. Some exercise beneficial but limits must be well defined. Keep warmly clad. Avoid chilling. Reduce if overweight. Take small meals of easily digested food. Rest immediately after meals. Take vasodilator drug before unavoidable exercise. Stop smoking. Beta-receptor blocking drugs very useful.

Myocardial infarction

Death of myocardium varying in extent depending on size of occluded artery.

Pathology. 1. Capillaries and venules of dead volume dilate and fill with stagnant blood.

2. Dead cells swell and soften (danger at this stage is that pressure inside ventricle during systole will be sufficient to burst myocardial wall).

3. Removal of all dead tissue and healing with fibrous tissue.

Signs and symptoms. Onset almost always suddenly while at rest. Similar distribution of pain to that of angina. Lasts for hours or days. Very severe, resistant to analgesics, even morphia.

Shock, due to generalised poor circulation following infarct: pallor, rapid shallow pulse, low blood pressure, subnormal temperature, nausea and vomiting, sometimes loss of consciousness.

Dyspnoea, fairly constant, due to engorgement of pulmonary vessels.

Cyanosis, not usually severe; face more ashen or leaden in hue. Sometimes atrial fibrillation; a bad sign if it occurs.

Diagnosis. ECG: Abnormal Q waves, elevated ST segment, later inversion of T waves.

Elevated levels of muscle enzymes in blood.

Creatine phosphokinase (CPK) rises within 12 hours. Lactic dehydrogenase (LDH) rises within 24 hours. Serum glutamic oxaloacetate (SGOT) rises last. Fall back to normal levels in same order. Can be used as measure of severity of infarction and of recovery.

Erythrocyte sedimentation rate (ESR) raised. Leucocytosis 10 000 to 20 000.

Course. 1. Death due to:

a. bursting of ventricle in soft state;

b. embolism from wall of ventricle affecting brain, kidney or further extending coronary blockage;

c. further extension of infarct due to added thrombosis.

d. interference with electric properties of myocardium.

2. Fairly rapid improvement. 2–3 weeks before good scar tissue formed and then return to fairly normal life.

3. Fairly rapid recovery but angina on exercise.

4. Congestive cardiac failure.

Best admitted to specialist unit with continuous monitoring facilities, and specialist staff. Ventricular fibrillation precedes sudden death in many cases. Suppression of myocardial irritability with lidocaine (Xylocaine) 50 to 100 mg i.v statim and 1 to 2 mg/minute as soon as ventricular premature beats detected.

Ventricular fibrillation needs immediate defibrillation. Atrial fibrillation less urgent but reduces cardiac efficiency and responds well to cardioversion when performed early.

Pain relieved with morphine sulphate 10 mg i.v. repeated in fifteen minutes and 3 to 4 hourly i.m. thereafter provided respiratory rate satisfactory. Meperidine (Pethidine) preferred by some. 50 mg i.v. or 100 mg i.m.

Rest essential. Absolute rest in bed for 3 to 4 days until danger of rupture of ventricle lessens. Thereafter careful introduction of self help programme. Sedation essential.

Oxygen often helpful in early stages especially if dyspnoea, cyanosis, shock and congestive failure present.

Anticoagulant therapy controversial, especially in mild cases. Initiated with heparin i.v. because of its immediate anticoagulant activity. 1000 units in 100 ml by burette per hour. Phenindione (Dindevan) 50 to 100 mg daily or dicoumarin (Warfarin) 3 to 10 mg daily for maintenance orally. Monitoring of prothrombin daily in early stages to establish requisite dose and weekly thereafter. Antidotes to anticoagulants, protamine sulphate 50 mg for heparin, vitamin K for phenindione and dicoumarin or transfusion of fresh whole blood.

Complications detected early and treated vigorously. Shock denoted by low systolic pressure and oliguria treated by inotropic agents — digitalis, isoprenalin. Jugular venous pressure monitored and fluid volume adjusted by i.v. fluids.

Congestive cardiac failure treated with diuretics, reduction of salt intake, and digitalisation — serum potassium monitored and maintained above 3·5 mmol/l by addition of potassium chloride to drip.

Heart block watched for especially in anterior infarction in which conduction system within septum involved. Indicated by lengthening of PR interval on ECG, dropped beats, dissociation of atrial and ventricular rates, Stokes-Adams attacks. Treated by transvenous pacemaker.

Atropine 0·6 to 1·2 mg i.v. blocks vagal influence and increases heart rate.

Rupture of septum tearing of leaflets of mitral valve or ventricular aneurysm may be amenable to surgery.

Rehabilitation. 2 to 3 weeks bed rest, 6 weeks of gradually increasing mobilization. 6 weeks of trial to establish residual function and accustom patient to a way of life best adapted to survival and optimum quality of life within limits set by condition.

Congestive cardiac failure

Myocardium fails to maintain onward flow of blood into pulmonary circulation, hold-up occurs throughout systemic veins.

Common causes. Coronary artery disease especially when right ventricle involved. Mitral stenosis because it holds up blood in lungs and throws a burden onto right ventricle. Rheumatic myocarditis. Hypertension. Pulmonary fibrotic disease. Congenital cardiac lesions. Syphilis.

Subdivisions. 1. Left ventricular failure (LVF) affects mainly respiratory system causing shortness of breath on exertion, nocturnal dyspnoea, orthopnoea, pulmonary venous congestion, cough.

2. Right ventricular failure (RVF) affects mainly systemic venous system causing raised jugular venous pressure, hepatomegaly, general oedema starting in dependent parts.

3. Mixed: Eventually either LVF or RVF takes on mixed pattern.

Stages. Back pressure in venae cavae causes hold-up of blood in all veins. All organs become engorged and their function impaired.

Brain. Throbbing headache. Blurred vision. Ringing noises in ears. Mental confusion, disorientation. Insomnia. Nightmares.

Liver. Engorgement and enlargement. Portal obstruction affecting all digestive organs: anorexia, nausea, vomiting, poor nutritional absorption, flatulence, constipation.

Kidneys. Diminished urinary output. Retention of salt and water hence generalised oedema with ascites and pleural effusion.

Lungs. Especially in mitral and aortic stenosis — dyspnoea, pulmonary oedema, haemoptysis, cyanosis.

Treatment. Depends on increasing heart's efficiency, reducing its work load, and getting rid of oedema. Rest. Digitalis. Diuretics. Diet. Rest under sedation in an upright position. Digitalis strengthens and slows heart beat and improves circulation generally. Uptake of oedema fluid and increased urinary output most beneficial. Diuretics, especially powerful ones — furosemide (Lasix) 40 to 80 mg i.v., i.m. or orally, ethacrynic acid (Edecrin) 25 to 100 mg orally, mercurials (Mersalyl) 1 ml i.m. two or three times a week.

Less powerful diuretics such as thiazides, or those with potassium sparing properties, e.g. aldosterone inhibitors (Aldactone), triamterine. [See p. 000]. Low serum potassium guarded against because of increased risk of digitalis toxicity.

Other means of removing fluid used if diuretics fail, peritoneal dialysis, paracentesis of chest or abdomen, rotating tourniquets, insertion of Southey's tubes. Aspiration of 200–500 ml ascitic fluid may initiate rapid absorption of remainder.

Diet should be light, easily digested and nourishing. Sometimes salt restricted until there is a good urinary flow. Fluid balance important and accurate charts should be kept.

Occasionally, especially if headache persistent, venesection performed, 500 ml of blood removed rapidly. Though this volume is made up by body very rapidly, patient often obtains relief for 2–3 months. Convalescence should be prolonged.

Prognosis. Treatment not curative. Condition progressive. Life lived so that no additional strain is put on heart. Weight controlled by careful dieting as lack of exercise and limitation of possibilities for active participation in most things leads easily to obesity.

Causes of CCF which may be curable are sought — mitral stenosis, some cases of coronary stenosis, valvular disease, myxoedema, anaemia, beri beri, thyrotoxicosis.

Hypertension

Blood pressure raised above 100 mmHg diastolic over age 50. Systolic pressure regarded with less significance than previously and may be above 150 without cause for alarm if diastolic remains below 90.

Types. Primary or essential hypertension. Secondary hypertension.

Primary hypertension

Cause unknown. Marked hereditary factor. More common in women.

Signs and symptoms. Steady rise in blood pressure starting at about 35–40 years of age. Pressure rarely greater than 200 systolic 110 diastolic. Often symptom free and remains undiscovered until patient attempts to become insured and condition discovered at medical examination.

Patients often of short thick-set build; red faced; energetic; capable personality.

Onset of complications may be first sign; cerebro-vascular accident, heart failure, epistaxis, failing vision.

Treatment. Avoidance of hard exercise, excitement, irritation, anger. Mild sedation, e.g. sodium amytal 30 mg thrice daily. Keep weight down a little below average for height and age. Antihypertensive drugs.

Secondary hypertension

Renal hypertension

When there is low blood pressure within the glomeruli a hormone [renin] similar in its effects to noradrenaline is released from kidney into general circulation, causing a marked rise in blood pressure. Renin is produced in chronic nephritis and in some cases of congenital stenosis of one renal artery. In the latter case nephrectomy cures the hypertension.

Phaeochromocytoma

A tumour of the adrenal gland causing oversecretion of adrenaline. The normal effect of adrenaline is accentuated — rapid pulse, faster, deeper respirations, blanched skin, slowed digestion, raised blood pressure. The latter may be continuous or it may occur paroxysmally.

Treatment, remove affected adrenal gland.

Toxaemia of pregnancy

Occurs after 28th week giving rise to high blood pressure, proteinuria and oedema. Rest may be enough if raised blood pressure occurs alone. If proteinuria and oedema occur patient should be admitted to hospital. High protein diet given for albumin loss; salt restricted to reduce oedema. Complications can be severe, e.g. eclampsia with convulsions and coma, retinal haemorrhage and blindness. Usually cured within 3 weeks of delivery.

High blood pressure in thyrotoxicosis
Slight rise usual; occasionally marked rise. Persists until endocrine imbalance corrected.

Malignant hypertension

Sudden rise of diastolic pressure to over 130 mmHg. Systolic pressure usually greater than 200.
Signs and symptoms. Severe headache, visual disturbance with papilloedema, retinal exudates and haemorrhages. Oliguria, blood and protein in urine. If untreated death often sudden from cardiac or renal failure or cerebro-vascular accident.
Pathology. Arteriolar necrosis, especially of glomerular vessels.
Treatment. Diazoxide (Hyperstat) 300 mg by very rapid i.v. injection, or pentolinium tartrate (Ansolysen) 1 to 2 mg i.m. hourly according to response, followed by beta adrenergic blocking agent or other maintenance anti-hypertensive.

Anti-hypertensive drugs

Chlorothiazide (Saluric. Chlotride)
Principally a diuretic which suppresses sodium reabsorption in kidney tubules. Moderate anti-hypertensive effect when given alone. Increases effect of other anti-hypertensives. Dosage as a diuretic — 0·5 to 2 g daily. As a co-hypotensive — 0·5 g daily. Side effects are electrolyte imbalance due to loss of sodium and potassium; may be necessary to give potassium chloride orally, or to conserve potassium with triamterene, amiloride or spironolactone.
Ganglion blocking agents (Hexamethonium. Pentolinium tartrate. Mecamylamine. Pentacynium).
Effect most profound when person standing. Dosage must be determined for each individual under medical supervision.

Tolerance develops to all, necessitating gradually increasing dosage until either their effect is negligible or until side effects are intolerable — mental depression; suicidal desires; Parkinsonism. Much less used than formerly.

Guanethedine sulphate (Ismelin)

A selective sympathetic inhibitor which does not affect parasympathetic system. Action is at neuro-muscular junction in arterioles blocking action of noradrenaline. Dosage — gradual increase from 10 mg daily at 4–6 days intervals, to 40–60 mg or higher daily. Side effects — dizziness, tiredness, faintness on standing, nasal stuffiness.

Alpha methyldopa (Aldomet)

Mode of action uncertain. Probably reduces sympathetic outflow from brain. Generally well tolerated. Side effects include postural hypotension, depression, drowsiness, dry mouth, haemolytic anaemia, liver dysfunction. Dosage — 500 to 2000 mg daily.

Beta adrenergic blocking drugs

Newer substances constantly appearing. Act by antagonising beta adrenergic effects. Beta receptors divided into beta 1 — cardiac: beta 2 — bronchial and arteriolar smooth muscle.

Blockade of beta 1 receptors slows heart rate, decreases contractility, slows conduction.

Blockade of beta 2 receptors constricts bronchioles, narrows arterioles.

Beta blockers divided into those acting on both receptor groups and those with relatively greater effect on beta one receptors i.e. those with cardioselectivity.

In latter group are:
    atenolol (Tenormin)
    metoprolol (Betaloc Lopresor)
Others acting on both receptors include:
    acebutolol
    alprenolol (Aptin. Betacard)
    oxprenolol (Trasicor)
    pindolol (Visken)
    propranolol (Inderal)

Increasing use in hypertension, angina, atrial and ventricular tachycardia, symptoms in hyperthyroid, phaeochromocytoma, migrain headache.

Contra indicated in heart failure, airways obstructive disease, and insulin dependent diabetes. Even the cardio selective blockers may cause difficulties in latter two classes of patients.

Probably drug of choice in hypertension. Dose varies with drug used. Most given once or twice daily. May be combined with other antihypertensive drugs.

Free from postural hypotension but care needed in presence of arteriosclerosis where some degree of hypertension necessary to maintain flow in extremities. May precipitate Raynaud's disease.

Clonidine (Catapres)

Acts centrally reducing sympathetic drive causing cardiac slowing and vasodilation. May react with other drugs having central activity e.g. alcohol, hypnotics, sedatives. May cause drowsiness, dry mouth, nausea, nightmares, Raynaud's phenomenon. Abrupt cessation of tablets may cause severe rebound hypertension.

Dosage — orally 75 mcg t.i.d. initially rising to 300 mcg t.i.d.

Hydrallazine (Apresoline)

Acts directly on arteriolar smooth muscle causing relaxation thus lowering peripheral resistance.

Generally used in conjunction with betablockers in cases where resistance to treatment occurs with betablockers alone. Hydrallazine alone induces reflex increase in heart rate and stroke volume and may precipitate angina, myocardial infarction, pulmonary hypertension in mitral valve incompetence, hence the need to prime patient with beta blockers.

Dose 50 mg daily increasing gradually to 200 mg daily.

Prazosin (Minipress)

Mode of action unknown. Causes peripheral vasodilation without reflex tachycardia. May be used alone for mild hypertension or in conjunction with other anti hypertensives in more severe cases.

Side effects include transitory dizziness, drowsiness, sweating, urinary frequency. Occasionally, headache, weakness, dry mouth, depression, vomiting and diarrhoea, pruritus and rash.

Dosage — 0·5 mg t.i.d. increasing slowly to effective dose up to 20 mg/day.

Diazoxide (Hyperstat)

Relaxes smooth muscle in peripheral arterioles reducing hypertension to normal levels within 5 minutes of intravenous administration and maintains reduction for several hours.

Used almost exclusively in dangerous hypertensive crises. i.v. bolus of 300 mg in 20 ml given quickly in 20 seconds, repeated 6 hourly if necessary.

Adverse reactions. Hypotension, nausea, vomiting, sensation of warm skin, headache.

Sodium Nitroprusside (Nipride)

Acts by relaxing peripheral arterioles. Effect is immediate on i.v. administration and ceases as soon as i.v. stopped. Useful in controlling dangerous hypertension while waiting for more sustained therapy to take effect.

Dosage 50 mg in i.l. 5 per cent dextrose given i.v. in 4 hours. Flask must be wrapped in foil to protect from light.

Congenital heart lesions

Patent ductus arteriosus

Persistence of ductus arteriosus during post-natal life. Ductus arteriosus is a normal structure during foetal life. Connects aorta and pulmonary artery to divert blood from pulmonary circulation. As soon as lungs inflate at birth, blood pressure in pulmonary artery falls. This allows ductus arteriosus to close in most cases. In a few it remains open.

Signs and symptoms. No symptoms where this is the only defect. Predisposition to bacterial endocarditis. Collapsing pulse (Corrigan's pulse). Stethescopically a continuous murmur can be heard as blood flows back from aorta into pulmonary artery. Radiographically pulmonary artery may be dilated and there may be some enlargement of left ventricle. Lung fields may appear denser on X-ray due to overfilling of pulmonary vessels.

Treatment. Ligation of ductus arteriosus.

Patent atrial foramen

Persistence of foramen ovale during post-natal life. The fora-men ovale is a natural opening between right and left atria during foetal life. Much of the blood entering right atrium is shunted directly to left atrium, so by-passing pulmonary circulation. As soon as lungs inflate at birth, pressure in right atrium falls lower than that in left atrium and this causes the membranous valve to close. It frequently remains open to a slight degree and seems to cause no disability whatsoever unless it is coupled with other congenital faults.

Signs and symptoms. Slight dyspnoea. X-ray shows enlarged atria; enlarged pulmonary arteries; overfilled lungs.

Complications. Interference with conducting mechanism — atrial fibrillation; heart block. Pulmonary embolism. Cerebral embolism from clot passing from right atrium through foramen into left side and hence into aorta. Pulmonary hypertension.

Treatment. None unless dyspnoea becomes severe, then surgical closure.

Ventricular septal defect

Persistent opening between ventricles due to failure of septum to complete its growth.

Signs and symptoms. Depends on size of opening. Small opening with normal pulmonary vascular resistance allows little shunting and no symptoms arise. Often this type produces a loud systolic murmur which is of no consequence whereas large defect with serious shunting may have soft almost inaudible murmur.

Signs of cardiac failure (LVF) when L to R shunting severe.

Treatment. If L to R shunting severe placement of band round pulmonary artery in early infancy may permit survival to an age when permanent closure may be performed. If severe L to R shunting continues unchecked, irreversible pulmonary hypertension results.

Prognosis. 30 per cent close spontaneously. 25 per cent develop pulmonary hypertension with clubbing of fingers and toes, polycythaemia and cyanosis.

Occasionally bacterial endocarditis develops. With large shunts congestive cardiac failure common.

Fallot's tetralogy

Four lesions occur simultaneously. In most cases the abnormalities are incompatible with life and the baby is either stillborn or dies shortly after birth. Even with lesser degrees where the baby is born alive, few live longer than 14 years unless surgery is possible.

Lesions: (1) Pulmonary stenosis; (2) hypertrophy of right ventricle; (3) interventricular septal opening; (4) aortic opening communicates with right ventricle as well as left.

Signs and symptoms. Extreme cyanosis due to large amount of deoxygenated blood passing from right ventricle back into general circulation without benefit of pulmonary refreshment. Dyspnoea severe especially on exertion. Child finds relief from dyspnoea by squatting. Fingers and toes clubbed. Polycythaemia — response to poor oxygenation of tissues. X-ray shows boot shaped heart ('coeur-en-sabot').

Treatment. Surgical closure of ventricular septal defect, especially if it can prevent communication between right atrium and aorta, brings great remission of symptoms. When inoperable — child raised in sheltered conditions where strain of any sort avoided. Other operations designed to improve pulmonary circulation but not to correct deformities — anastomosis of left subclavian artery to pulmonary artery; anastomosis between aorta and pulmonary artery; valvotomy of pulmonary valve.

Eisenmenger's syndrome

Formerly defined as combination of ventricular septal defect, right ventricular hypertrophy, overriding aorta. Now accepted as any case in which a former left to right shunt has reversed direction of flow owing to increased pulmonary hypertension.

May occur in ventricular septal defect, atrial septal defect, patent ductus arteriosus.

Signs and symptoms. Exertional dyspnoea. Cyanosis. Clubbing. Polycythaemia. Right ventricular heave. Systolic murmur X-ray shows enlarged pulmonary arteries.

Prognosis. Death from congestive cardiac failure. Thrombosis.

Coarctation of the aorta

Constriction of aorta just beyond the branching off of left subclavian artery.

Signs and symptoms. Dilatation of other arteries provide collateral supply of blood to parts of body distal to constriction, especially internal mammary arteries, intercostal arteries and branches of subclavian arteries. Blood pressure raised in upper part of body, decreased or absent in lower parts.

Prognosis. Hypertension, cerebral haemorrhage, bacterial endocarditis, occur if not corrected.

Treatment. Resection of affected part and anastomosis. Teflon replacement may be necessary.

Aneurysm

A dilation in the walls of an artery. Most often associated with arteriosclerosis.

Types. Syphilitic; dissecting; congenital.

Syphilitic aneurysm

An occurrence in third stage syphilis in which tunica media destroyed and replaced with fibrous tissue. Owing to high blood pressure in arteries the fibrous section balloons and may burst.

Site. Most commonly arch of aorta; occasionally branches of the arch; less commonly thoracic or abdominal parts of aorta.

Signs and symptoms. Nil until aneurysm presses on nearby structures then depends on which structures are involved: (1) recurrent laryngeal nerve — hoarseness of voice and brassy cough; (2) bronchus — cough; later — bronchiectasis, sputum retention, atelectasis; (3) sternum — pain, erosion, pulsating swelling under skin; (4) on vertebrae — pain, collapse of vertebrae and kyphosis, pressure on cord with paraplegia; (5) oesophagus — dysphagia. Often associated with arotic valve incompetence — collapsing (waterhammer, Corrigan's) pulse.

Termination. Cardiac failure. Rupture and death by rapid haemorrhage.

Treatment. Treatment of underlying syphilis. This will prevent further destruction of tissue but has no effect on damage done. Avoid anything which may raise blood pressure — worry, anger, temper, excitement, over exertion. Surgical removal of aneurysm and replacement with teflon graft.

Dissecting aneurysm

Through a weak point in the intima blood penetrates between

it and tunica media, thus creating a false passage. Atheroma and hypertension often present. Patient usually over 60 years.

Signs and symptoms. Severe thoracic, back or abdominal pain. Shock, Occlusion of one or more branches of aorta may occur — hence, depending on which vessels are blocked, syncope, loss of one or both radial pulses, paraplegia from loss of blood supply to spinal cord via intercostal arteries. If aorta ruptures sudden death may occur. Confirmation of diagnosis may be revealed by angiography showing a 'double-barrelled' appearance of aorta.

Treatment. Absolute rest in bed. Treat shock. Lower blood pressure. Later — surgery. Resection of part with replacement by grafting.

Congenital aneurysm (Berry aneurysm)

Small aneurysm projects from circle of Willis or from its branches. Size varies from pin head to pea. No symptoms unless it bursts then signs and symptoms of sub-arachnoid haemorrhage. Rare before age 40.

Symptoms. Similar to meningitis, sudden severe headache, may follow escape of blood into theca — rigidity of neck and back muscles; positive Kernig's sign; cerebro-spinal fluid red or bright yellow xanthocromia.

Treatment. Absolute rest for one month to allow clot to organise in aneurysm. Lumbar puncture to reduce intracranial pressure, because of high risk of recurrence. Attempts may be made to tie off aneurysm. Common carotid artery may be tied off after ascertaining position of aneurysm by arteriogram. Experimental — obliteration of aneurysm by insertion of special needle through which liquid helium can be introduced (cryosurgery). Metal clips placed across neck of aneurysm.

Other common sites of aneurysm

Abdominal aorta. Femoral, popliteal arteries.

Abdominal aorta. Almost always below origin of renal arteries.

Signs and symptoms. None during early stages.

Pulsatile swelling found during abdominal examination or calcification in walls seen on X-ray. Later pressure on surrounding structure causes pain. Thrombi from wall may dislodge and cause blockage distally. Rupture may occur at any time. May be catastrophic but often slow persistent bleeding into retroperitoneal tissues may give time for diagnosis and treatment.

Treatment. Surgical removal of dilated portion of aorta and iliac arteries and replacement with Dacron graft.

Femoral and popliteal arteries.

Usually arteriosclerotic. Often bilateral. Easily diagnosed — pulsatile swelling readily palpable. Occasionally thrombosis fills aneurysm which stops pulsating and pain, pallor, numbness and gangrene may occur.

Treatment. Replacement of aneurysm with Dacron graft or ligation above and below with bypass.

Raynaud's disease

Vascular spasm resulting in ischaemia, usually of hands, in response to cold. Normal skin reaction to cold is blanching due to contraction of skin vessels, then dilatation with reddening of skin and increased circulation. In susceptible people constriction of vessels is intense and prolonged.

Aetiology. Usually an inherited condition. Only occurs in cold climates. More common in females. Starts in early adult life but no age exempt. *Stages*. 1. Spasm of arterioles producing pallor and numbness.

2. Local anoxia with cyanosis and pain.

3. Relaxation of arterioles with hyperaemia — red, swollen, intensely painful. Occasionally — no relaxation, gangrene.

Treatment. Mainly preventive. Avoid cold by staying in warm atmosphere. If impossible, don warmed clothing before exposure to cold. Don well fitting gloves — cotton next to skin, then wollen, then fur or leather if exposure prolonged or intense.

During attack — wrap part to protect from injury and wait for dilatation of skin vessels. Do not apply extra warmth or immerse in warm water. Cervical sympathetic ganglionectomy gives marked relief but condition recurs.

Thrombo-angiitis obliterans (Buerger's disease)

Endarteritis causing thickening of tunica intima of arteries of legs with consequent reduction of blood supply to feet and toes. Gangrene may result.

Signs and symptoms. Persistent coldness of feet. Diminished or absent pulse in dorsalis pedis artery. Intermittent claudication (anoxia of calf muscles causing spasm and severe pain when walking). Superficial venous thrombosis.

Treatment. Alternate raising and lowering of limb for 5 minute intervals continued for half an hour 4 or 5 times a day. Remain in warm environment. Wear warm clothing. Surgical replacement of affected vessel with graft. Lumbar sympathectomy tried but not always or permanently effective. Patient must stop smoking.

Care of gangrenous limb

Prevention most important. Often starts with minor trauma especially in elderly patients with arteriosclerosis — stubbing toe, ill fitting shoes, shrunken socks, inexpert attention to corn. Keep part dry, immobile and cool with good circulation of air all round. Line of demarcation between healthy and gangrenous tissue clearly defined. If circulation up to this line satisfactory, and if sepsis can be avoided, the gangrenous part will mummify and separate. If sepsis occurs, toxic absorption causes severe general reaction; death rate high. Hence need for careful observation to detect sepsis early enough for amputation before severe toxaemia.

Great care and attention must be paid to sound limb in all cases of gangrene so that patient has every chance of early rehabilitation if amputation becomes necessary.

Diseases of venous system

Varicose veins

Dilated, tortuous veins with inefficient valves. Most commonly affect superficial veins of legs — long and short saphenous veins and their branches. Often perforating veins linking superficial and deep systems are inefficient allowing reflux of blood from deep system.

Causes and contributing factors. Hereditary weakness. Prolonged standing. Pregnancy. Valve damage due to thrombosis.

Signs and symptoms. May be entirely symptomless. Aching

after standing. Muscular cramps. Dermatitis. Atrophy of skin of lower leg. Brown pigmentation. Ulceration.

Trendelenburgh's Test. Patient placed supine with leg elevated until veins empty. Tourniquet placed round thigh. Patient stands and veins observed for method of filling. Rapid filling indicates incompetent perforating veins. Lower placement of tourniquet at successive levels can place accurately site of incompetent perforators.

Treatment. Medical. Support with elastic stockings. Elevation of legs as frequently as possible. Avoid long standing. Avoid trauma. *Surgical*: Injection of sclerosing agents to cause thrombosis of short segments for mild disease. For more severe cases stripping of main vessel, ligation of collaterals and obliteration of perforators. Early ambulation post operatively.

Complications. Development of ulcer, spontaneously or secondary to trauma. Rupture of varicosities with severe haemorrhage. Thrombophlebitis. Stasis dermatitis.

Thrombophlebitis. A. Superficial

Inflammation along course of superficial vein. May be spontaneous or secondary to trauma, intravenous catheterisation; carcinoma of pancreas, pregnancy.

Signs and symptoms. Painful limb, tenderness along course of affected vessel. Inflammation, swelling.

Treatment. Rest with leg elevated. Local warmth. Anti-inflammatory drugs, indomethacin [Indocid], phenylbutazone [BTZ], aspirin. Ligation of vein at junction with deep vessels. Anticoagulants if extension into deep vessels occurs.

B. Deep

Thrombosis with secondary inflammation of vessel, occurring most frequently postoperatively, post-partum, post-trauma, and in CCF, myocardial infarction, endocarditis.

Almost always of calf vessels or venous lakes of gastrocnemius and soleus muscles. Usually history of circulatory stasis, pressure on calf, chronic infection. Other contributory factors — shock, hypotension, anaemia, leukaemia or other malignancy.

Pathology. Increased platelet cohesiveness allows micro-clots to form in static blood pools. These act as nuclei for fibrin deposition and red cell coagulation. Once lumen blocked clot formation extends proximally into other veins.

Signs and symptoms. May be none until pulmonary embolus occurs with cough, chest pain, dyspnoea, sputum and haemoptysis. Often pain in calf especially when foot is dorsiflexed (Homan's sign). Ankle oedema, cyanosis of limb. Diagnosis by phlebography, presence of fibrinogen degradation products in circulating blood, raised white cell count.

Prevention. Avoid pressure on calves in bed or on theatre table. Electrical stimulation of calf muscles during operation to prevent stasis. Subcutaneous injection of low dose calcium heparin 5000 units 12 hourly pre-operatively for 3 or 4 days, and after first post-operative day. Early ambulation. Aspirin 1 g daily to reduce platelet adhesiveness.

Treatment. Anticoagulation using heparin initially 10 000 to 30 000 units daily i.v. continuous drip for 3 days overlapped by oral warfarin or phenindione according to prothrombin time.

Streptokinase i.v. used to dissolve existing clots and pulmonary emboli.

Elastic stocking applied to affected limb. Leg elevated 15 degrees. Exercise encouraged when inflammation and oedema subside.

If pulmonary emboli recur, ligation of femoral vein or fenestration of inferior vena cava.

Pulmonary embolism. (See p. 58).

Diseases of red blood cells: *Anaemia*

Reduction in quantity or quality of circulating erythrocytes. *Terms used.* Normocytic — circulating erythrocytes of normal size and shape. Microcytic — erythrocytes smaller than normal. Macrocytic — erythrocytes larger than normal. Megalocytic — immature erythrocytes larger than normal in circulation. Normochromic — normal redness of erythrocytes when compared to a standard. Hypochromic — erythrocytes paler than normal. Hyperchromic — erythrocytes more deeply coloured than normal.

Classification of anaemia. (1) Haemorrhagic (a) acute, (b) chronic; (2) Haemolytic; (3) Dietetic; (4) Haemopoietic.

Acute haemorrhagic anaemia

Causes. Trauma or disease (haemoptysis, haematemesis, haematuria etc.).

Signs and symptoms. Obvious bleeding if external. If concealed (haemothorax, haemoperitoneum) — skin pale, cold, clammy; pulse rapid, thready; respirations rapid and shallow at first, deep and sighing later due to general anoxia; temperature normal at first, later subnormal; blood pressure falls rapidly, dangerous below 90 mmHg systolic; mental symptoms due to hypoxia — restlessness, giddiness, faintness, later — dim vision, ringing noises in head, unconsciousness. Blood changes — none at first then low haemoglobin and low haematocrit as blood volume is made up with water, either from drinking or from tissue fluid.

Treatment. Depends on cause and amount lost. If 600 ml or less (blood donor) rest for one hour, allay thirst, increase iron intake for one month. If more than 600 ml — put to bed with foot of bed elevated. Allay thirst. Blood transfusion, equivalent in amount to that lost. Morphine to ease restlessness. Treat cause.

Chronic haemorrhagic anaemia

Cause. Continuous or frequent small haemorrhages depleting circulating blood faster than production can replace it. Constant loss of iron depletes liver's stores rapidly, hence haemoglobin manufacture held up. Commonly occurs in duodenal ulcer, haemorrhoids, intestinal cancer, hookworm infestation, scurvy.

Signs and symptoms. Few until anaemia severe. Increasing weakness; rapid fatigue on exercise; increasing pallor; giddiness; syncope; headache; shortness of temper; irregular menstruation or amenorrhoea; rapid pulse; reduced blood pressure. Erythrocytes — hypochromic; microcytic. Haemoglobin — lowered; may be very low — 20 per cent. Bone marrow — hyperplasia (excessive formation of erythroblasts).

Treatment. Diagnose and treat cause. Treat anaemia with transfusion of packed cells if erythrocyte count below 3½ million. Give iron (p. 35).

Haemolytic anaemia

Cause. Breakdown of erythrocytes faster than production. Cause of breakdown may be: (1) mechanical — malaria parasites invade erythrocytes, multiply, break out and invade new cells. (2) Toxic — toxin of haemolytic streptococci destroys cell membrane. Some drugs, e.g. trinitrotoluene, render cells more fragile and subject to rapid breakdown. (3) Splenic — spleen becomes overactive.

Special types. Congenital (familial microcytosis). Erythrocytes small, spherical, extremely fragile. Spleen and liver enlarged. Jaundice present. Gallstones present in 60 per cent of cases.

Treatment. Splenectomy at 10 years of age.

Erythroblastosis foetalis. Mother develops antibodies to child's erythrocytes. Antibodies cross placenta into child's blood stream and destroy its erythrocytes. Usually mother Rhesus negative and child Rhesus positive (p. 47). First child usually born alive but jaundiced. Second and subsequent pregnancies reinforce production of antibodies and child stillborn. Greatest danger to child is permanent brain damage from presence of abnormal quantities of bilirubin. Treatment aimed at reducing bilirubin below danger level by exchange transfusion. Immunization of women at risk now possible.

Dietetic anaemia: Pernicious anaemia. Cause. Lack of circulating vitamin B_{12} due to absence of intrinsic factor in gastric juice. Lack of intrinsic factor may be congenital or due to gastrectomy or secondary to gastric disease, e.g. carcinoma. Vitamin B_{12} and folic acid are interrelated in their action in an unknown way.

Signs and symptoms. Onset most common in 40–60 age group. Gradually increasing muscular weakness; early onset of fatigue and dyspnoea on exercise; increasing pallor with a faint yellowish tinge; rapid pulse; tongue smooth, devoid of papillae and often sore; *Blood picture*. Erythrocytes of varying sizes mostly macrocytic; in untreated cases erythrocyte count may fall to 1 million per mm³; reticulocytes and normoblasts present in circulating blood; white cells and platelets also reduced.

Nerve complication. Vitamin B_{12} also needed by nerve cells especially in spinal cord. Prolonged lack of vitamin B_{12} causes irreversible degeneration of axon cylinders resulting in failure to transmit impulses. Result — combined acute degeneration of spinal cord with partial paralysis, tingling, pins and needles and anaesthesia of skin especially of lower limbs.

Diagnosis. Full blood examination. Fractional test meal reveals complete absence of hydrochloric acid (achlorhydria). Examination of red marrow shows many enlarged nucleated red cells (megaloblasts) and scanty normoblasts. Hypersegmented ploymorphs.

Serum B_{12} level reduced to below 100 pg/ml. [N-300 to 400 pg/ml). Schilling test proves reduced intestinal absorption of B_{12}.Radioactive labelled B_{12} 0·5 micrograms given orally. Two hours later 1 mg unlabelled B_{12} given i.m. Urinary and faecal excretion then measured.

In pernicious anaemia urinary excertion of radioactive B_{12} reduced to 5 per cent or less of administered dose while faecal excretion remains high. Simultaneous administration of intrinsic factor alters absorption to normal.

Treatment. Immediate transfusion of packed cells if erythrocyte count below 3½ million. Large initial injections of vitamin B_{12} — up to 1000 micrograms twice weekly — until erythrocyte count normal, then maintenance dose 50–100 mcg monthly. If subacute combined degeneration also present large doses may be continued for as long as 6 months.

Iron deficiency anaemia

A microcytic, hypochromic anaemia due to insufficient iron.

Causes. Lack of iron may be due to a number of causes — insufficient iron in diet; loss of iron in haemorrhage especially chronic haemorrhage; fetal demands on mother; deficient absorption due to any form of intenstinal hurry; failure to utilise available iron, e.g. in cancer, tuberculosis, nephritis; lack of hydrochloric acid in gastric juice to convert ferric compounds to ferrous compounds, only the latter being absorbed from intestines.

Signs and symptoms. Reduced oxygen-carrying power of erythrocytes responsible for symptoms even when erythrocyte count normal. Tiredness; rapid onset of fatigue and dyspnoea on exercise; pallor of skin and mucous membranes; skin dry and scaly; nails brittle and spoon-shaped.

Serum iron reduces to ⅓ normal or less. Iron binding capacity increased. Marrow haemosiderin absent. Normoblasts plentiful.

Treatment. Administer iron: (1) *Orally*. Many preparations available. Ferrous sulphate (Fersolate) 1 tablet (200 mg) 3 times daily. Ferrous carbonate (Blaud's pill) 3 g daily. Disadvantages: Iron salts irritate gastric mucosa causing dyspepsia. Liquid preparations stain teeth. Sometimes cause diarrhoea, sometimes constipation. Toxic to children even in small doses. Absorption variable but always small. (2) *Intramuscularly*. Iron — dextran complex (Imferon) 50–100 mg twice weekly until haemoglobin normal.

Disadvantages: Must be given deeply into large muscle. Pain and staining of skin if given shallowly. (3) *Intravenously*. Saccharated iron oxide (Ferrivenin) 100 mg in 5 ml on alternate days. Each injection raises haemoglobin by 4 per cent. Disadvantages: Possibility of general reaction. Hence test dose given first — 1 ml. If no reaction within half an hour remainder given. Possible reactions — dizziness, nausea, pain in abdomen. Each injection given very slowly to avoid local pain along course of vein and thrombophlebitis. Patient kept under observation throughout course.

Folic acid deficiency

Mimics pernicious anemia.

Causes. Inadequate intake. More rapid utilization. Interference with folic acid metabolism. Arises in association with alcoholism, pregnancy, malabsorption, certain drug treatment — anticonvulsants and certain cytotoxics which interfere with folate metabolism — methotrexate, pyrimethamine, triamterene.

Signs and symptoms. As for other anaemias.

Diagnosis. Low serum folate activity less then ½ normal. Hypersegmented polymorphs. Megaloblastic marrow.

Treatment. Oral folic acid 5 mg daily.

Haemopoietic anaemia

Anaemia due to destruction, derangement or replacement of haemocytoblasts (aplastic anaemia).

Causes. (1) Idiopathic; (2) poisoning by various drugs — phenylbutazone, benzol, arsenic, gold, sulphonamides, amidopyrine; (3) exposure to radioactive substances — X-rays, gamma rays from radium, cobalt or any source of radioactivity; (4) bacterial toxins — diphtheria; (5) exhaustion of bone marrow due to overproduction for many years — polycythaemia; (6) replacement by abnormal marrow — leukaemia, neoplasm.

Signs and symptoms. Depends on severity. Usually associated with reduction in leucocytes and platelets. Hence tendency to infections, capillary haemorrhages. Increasing pallor, tiredness, breathlessness.

Treatment. Search for cause. Discontinue current drug therapy. Administer androgenic steroids to stimulate marrow, testosterone enanthate 200 to 400 mg/kg twice weekly, nandrolone decanoate 1·5 mg/kg weekly. Platelet transfusion may reverse bleeding tendency. Splenectomy may slow down red cell destruction. Marrow transplant becoming possible. Repeated transfusions may prolong life.

Prognosis. Depends on severity and cause. Sometimes spontaneous recovery if recognised early and cause removed.

Polycythaemia

An increase in the number of circulating erythrocytes.

Types. (1) Polycythaemia vera. (2) Secondary consequent to oxygen want.

Polycythaemia vera

Cause unknown. Erythrocytes increased up to 11 million per mm^3. Leucocytes and platelets increased in proportion.

Signs and symptoms. Headache; giddiness; fainting; plum coloured facies; acne; pain in bones sometimes severe; enlarged spleen and liver. Thrombosis common due to high blood viscosity. Death often due to coronary or cerebral thrombosis.

Treatment. Temporary relief — venesection, 600 ml removed gives some symptomatic relief for 2–3 months. Suppression of bone marrow with radioactive agents or with cytotoxic drugs. Single injection of radio-active phosphorus, P^{32}, 3·8 millicuries. Whole body irradiation with X-rays. Nitrogen mustard 0·1 mg per kg body weight daily for 6 days.

Secondary polycythaemia

Normal response to low level of circulating oxygen or when extra demands for oxygen are made. Occurs in trained athletes, persons living at great heights above sea level, persons with impaired respiratory surface, e.g. emphysema, pulmonary fibrosis, and in heart lesions where blood is shunted from right to left side of heart without sufficient passing through lungs, e.g. Fallot's tetralogy. White cells and platelets remain normal.

Thalassaemia (Cooley's anaemia)

An inherited haemolytic anaemia occurring most commonly in

persons of Mediterranean descent. Autosomal recessive: Abnormal haemoglobin formed in reduced quantities. If defective gene inherited from one parent only (heterozygous) thalassaemia minor results — a mild anaemia often symptomless. If from both parents (homozygous) thalassaemia major with fatal outcome in teens at least.

Blood picture. Minor: Raised red cell count with thin cells — target cells. Great variation in red cell size (poikilocytosis). Stippling of red cells. Increased reticulocytes. Alteration in electrophoretic pattern of haemoglobin depending on type of abnormality — usually increased fetal haemoglobin level, increased haemoglobin A2.

May be mistaken for iron deficiency picture but marrow haemosiderin always present and anaemia does not respond to treatment with iron.

Major: Severe anaemia starting in early childhood. Hepato-splenomegaly.

Signs and symptoms. Pallor, failure to thrive, pot belly.

Severe anaemia with microcystosis and hypochromia. Raised serum bilirubin. Vast increases in foetal haemoglobin. Skull X-ray shows widening of medulla and thinning of cortex of bones producing diagnostic 'hair on end' picture.

Treatment. Of minor — none needed. Of major — repeated transfusions. Splenectomy if secondary haemolytic anaemia makes condition worse. Iron overloading from transfusion leads to iron deposition in all tissues which eventually interferes with function of heart, liver, pancreas. This effect partly reduced by transfusing frozen erythrocytes and by using chelating agents such as desferrioxamine or diethlene-triaminopenta acetate.

Sickle cell anaemia

An inherited haemolytic anaemia in which the haemoglobin molecule is abnormal. Cells containing this type of haemoglobin assume a sickle shape when deoxygenated. Confined to persons of Negro descent. Not incompatible with life and health when inherited from one parent only.

Moderate anaemia present all the time. Increased reticulocytes. Moderate jaundice.

Sickle cell crises. Whenever conditions favour deoxygenation sickling occurs. Blood becomes viscous causing small vessel blockages giving rise to severe bone and joint pain, tender rigid abdomen often mistakenly diagnosed as perforated ulcer or appendicitis, thrombosis of cerebral, pulmonary, mesenteric, splenic, renal vessels.

Treatment. Oxygen. Transfusion. Treat infections vigorously.

Other types of anaemia arise secondary to diseases, e.g. common accompaniment to cancer, chronic infection, cirrhosis, uraemia.

Treatment is of underlying disease.

Diseases of white cells: Agranulocytosis

Reduction in number of circulating granulocytes.

Causes. Destruction of parent cells in bone marrow by: (1) drugs — chloramphenicol, sulphonamides, thiouracil, amido-pyrine, butazolidine; (2) Gamma radiation — radioactive substances, radium, isotopes, X-rays, atomic piles.

Signs and symptoms. Rapid onset of severe infections of mucous membranes especially of mouth, throat, respiratory tract, gastro-intestinal tract.

Treatment. Immediate cessation of causative agent. Large doses of penicillin, especially methicillin which is effective against penicillin-resistant strains of staphylococci. Isolation of patient from sources of infection — limit number of attendants, who should be masked, gowned and gloved; sterilize room and contents; use sterilized bed linen; bar visitors from inside room. Take especial care of skin to prevent infections.

Prognosis. Depends on early diagnosis, hence need for white cell count immediately patient complains of sore throat when receiving drugs of risk mentioned previously. Often rapidly fatal but possible for marrow to regenerate.

Leukaemia

Malignant change in parent cells of either leucocytes or lymphocytes in which circulatory system flooded with immature white cells. Secondary anaemia due to crowding out of erythroblasts. Cause unknown.

Types: 1. Myeloid leukaemia (a) acute; (b) chronic.
2. Lymphocytic leukaemia (a) acute; (b) chronic.

3. Acute monocytic leukaemia.

The acute varieties are similar to each other and often difficult to distinguish.

Acute leukaemias

Signs and symptoms. Pallor due to anaemia; haemorrhages varying in degree from purpuric spots to frank bleeding from gums, nose, rectum or uterus; ulceration, sometimes severe, of gums, cheeks, tonsils; enlargement of lymph nodes; enlarged spleen; enlarged liver; pain in bones; temperature usually elevated to 30–40°C.

Diagnosis. White cell count elevated often to 100 000 per mm^3. Occasionally abnormal white cells retained in marrow and not found in circulating blood — aleukaemic leukaemia.

Treatment. Transfusion of fresh blood may give temporary improvement. Antibiotics to combat infection. Combinations of cytotoxic agents destroy leukaemic cells at various stages of their growth and maturation, vincristine during mitosis, mercaptopurine during DNA synthesis, methotrexate and cyclophosphamide during protein synthesis, prednisolone kills blast cells, radiation attacks cells protected by blood-brain barrier within CNS. Other cytotoxics — arabinoside, daunorubicin, thioguanine.

Long remission of symptoms achieved by repeated courses. A few cures claimed.

Complications from powerful drugs inevitable, lowered resistance to infections from organisms not usually pathogenic, needing i.v. antibiotics. Bleeding needing platelet transfusion. Gout from high levels of uric acid needing allopurinol (Zyloprim) 200 mg tds.

Recently, good results achieved by stimulation of immune process with BCG vaccine and snap-frozen irradiated leukaemic cells.

Chronic myeloid leukaemia

A leukaemia characterised by an increase in immature leucocytes to as much as 100 000 per mm^3 with splenomegaly and hepatomegaly, running fatal course of 1–5 years.

Treatment. Aim is to reduce leucocyte count to below 20 000. The following may be used:

Whole body irradiation with X-rays. Local irradiation to

spleen, liver or lymph nodes. Radioactive phosphorus. P^{32} given in carefully measured doses at 2 week intervals until reduction of leucocytes occurs, and maintenance doses every 1–3 months. Busulphan (Myleran), 4 mg daily for 8–12 weeks with smaller maintenance doses thereafter. Chorambucil (Leukeran) 0·1 mg/kg.

Chronic lymphocytic leukaemia

A leukaemia characterised by enlargement of all lymphoid tissue with white cell counts up to 100 000 mm³ — mostly lymphocytes. Duration: 3–20 years. Occurs most commonly in people over 40 years. Males 4 times more commonly than females.

Treatment. Similar to above.

Hodgkin's disease

Progressive disease characterised by painless enlargement of lymphoid tissue with weight loss, fever and anaemia.

Signs and symptoms. No age immune but characteristically male about 30 years. Insidious onset with one or more groups of lymph nodes swollen and painless. Enlarged spleen. Occasionally enlarged liver. Temperature raised, often in recurrent bouts lasting 10–14 days with remission for 10–14 days between. Enlarged nodes may become massive and cause pressure symptoms. Depending on site — trachea, bronchus, oesophagus, brachial plexus, recurrent laryngeal nerve, spinal nerves. Progressive anaemia.

Diagnosis and staging. Blood examination shows lymphocytopenia. Lymph node biopsy show abnormal proliferation of lymphocytes, histiocytes and Reed-Sternberg giant cells. Severity of disease determined prior to treatment.

Stage 0. Diagnosis from biopsy of node without symptoms.

Stage 1. One node only affected.

Stage 2. More than one node all above or all below diaphragm.

Stage 3. Nodes above and below diaphragm but no other tissues affected.

Stage 4. Other tissues involved — bone, marrow, lungs, liver, kidney, CNS.

Treatment. Depends on stage. Stages 1, 2, 3 — radiation may totally irradicate disease especially stages 1 and 2.

Combined chemotherapy in Stage 4 produces long periods of remission. Many schemes in use, e.g. MOPP mechlorethamine, oncovin, procarbazine, prednisolone. Careful calculation of dosage and time of administration. Observation for complications and side effects. Assessment of effectiveness.

Mechlorethamine (Mustagen) 0.4 mg/kg given i.v. while fasting. Nausea and vomiting controlled with antiemetics. Chlorambucil (Leukeran) 0.2 mg/kg in divided doses. Side effects rare. Vincristine (Oncovin) 0.1 mg/kg i.v. weekly. Procarbazine 50–200 mg orally daily. Prednisolone 50–60 mg daily. Intermittent courses of 14 days duration with 14 days between.

Other cytotoxics — cyclophosphamide, vinblastine, bleomycin.

Patient should be encouraged to carry on a normal life for as long as possible. Eventually, anaemia and weakness necessitate complete bed rest and nursing skill needed to prevent pressure sores and maintain morale.

Multiple myeloma

Malignant disease of plasma cells which produce immunoglobulins (Ig). Normal Ig molecules composed of 4 polypeptide chains, 2 light chains similar in all forms of Ig and 2 heavy chains different in each class of Ig. Light and heavy chain production balances except in multiple myeloma. Usually excessive light chains produced and insufficient normal Ig synthesised. Rarely heavy chains produced in excess.

Signs and symptoms. Anaemia. Bone pain especially when in motion. Spontaneous fractures. Very high ESR. Marked rouleau formation. Serum globulin greatly increased. Bence-Jones protein in urine in 40 per cent of cases — double light chains which solidify when urine heated and liquefy again when urine boiled. Electrophoresis of plasma shows peak of gamma globulins. X-ray shows circular, punched out, areas widely scattered throughout affected bones. Amyloid deposits throughout many organs interferes with functions causing weakness, weight loss, infections.

Treatment. Palliative only. Keep patient mobile. Maintain fluid intake to prevent renal failure due to protein deposition. Analgesics and irradiation for bone pain, gamma-globulin and antibiotics to combat infection. Disappointing results from cytotoxic drugs.

Prognosis. Some patients reach stable phase and survive for many years. Average survival from diagnosis 2 years.

Myelofibrosis
Progressive fibrosis of marrow displacing haemopoietic tissue. Often end result of myeloid leukaemia, polycythaemia, metastatic carcinoma.

Signs and symptoms. Increasing weakness, weight loss, pancytopenia, splenomegaly, hepatomegaly. Marrow often impossible to obtain by sternal aspiration and biopsy necessary. Red cells have bizarre shapes. Raised serum alkaline phosphatase. Early platelet increase, later greatly diminished.

Treatment. Transfusion. Stimulation of existing bone marrow with androgens. Splenectomy.

Diseases of blood platelets: thrombocytopenia

Reduction in number of circulating platelets.
Causes. 1. Primary. Cause unknown but splenectomy sometimes cures.

2. Secondary (a) accompanying aplastic anaemia; (b) accompanying toxic states — some drugs, bacterial toxins.

Signs and symptoms. Increased permeability of capillaries; haemorrhages into skin, mucous membranes, nephrons, retina, endometrium, joints. Bleeding time increased (Duke's test — skin is pricked and blood continuously removed with absorbent paper until it ceases to flow. Normal 3–5 minutes). Hess's test positive (tourniquet applied to limb with sufficient pressure to occlude superficial veins — 80 mmHg. Petechiae appear distal to tourniquet within 2–3 minutes).

Treatment. Depends on severity. None in mild cases. Splenectomy in severe primary condition. Blood transfusion in severe haemorrhage with anaemia. Treat underlying cause in secondary type.

Haemophilia

Haemorrhagic disease caused by lack of antihaemophilic

globulin (Factor VIII). Females transmit the disease but do not usually suffer from it.

Pathology. Sex determined at moment of conception. Ova possess one X chromosome, spermatozoa possess either an X or a Y chromosome. If an X-bearing sperm unites with an ovum, offspring female. If a Y-bearing sperm unites with an ovum, offspring male. Gene for haemophilia carried on X chromosome and is recessive. In females carrying haemophiliac gene the effects are cancelled by the other X chromosome and the female does not suffer from haemophilia, but can transmit it to her sons. In males who inherit the gene for haemophilia with the X chromosome from their mother, there is no counterbalancing gene in the Y chromosome from their father hence such males suffer from haemophilia.

Signs and symptoms. Prolonged clotting time: 1–12 hours. Haemorrhages, especially after trivial injuries. (Ability to form *plasma* thrombokinase impaired by absence of antihaemophilic globulin, hence minor injuries result in prolonged bleeding. Ability to produce *tissue* thrombokinase not impaired, hence major trauma with severe damage to tissues produces sufficient thrombokinase for clotting to occur).

Treatment. If patient is to survive childhood great vigilance needed to prevent minor injuries. Haemorrhage can be stopped by (1) transfusion of normal blood, (2) intravenous injection of antihaemophilic globulin, (3) local application of substances rich in thrombokinase, e.g. Russell's viper venom.

Vitamin K deficiency

Prothrombin essential for blood clotting. Produced in liver in presence of vitamin K. Vitamin K absorbed from intestines only if bile salts present, hence absence of bile, due either to obstructive jaundice or to hepatitis, results in insufficient vitamin K absorption, reduced prothrombin production, prolonged clotting time and haemorrhage. Treatment, especially when surgery is contemplated, involves supplying vitamin K either directly by injection or indirectly by feeding the patient bile salts.

Prothrombin time. A test which indirectly reveals amount of prothrombin in blood. Sample of oxalated blood collected. To this, all the factors needed to bring about clotting except prothrombin are added. Time taken for clot to form therefore dependent on amount of prothrombin present. Normal time: 10–12 seconds.

Intravascular clotting (thrombosis)

Anything inside blood vessels which destroys negative charge of lining membrane causes platelets to adhere to wall and break down thus liberating cephalins for formation of thrombokinase.

Causes. Atheromatous plaques; stasis of blood due to pressure; low blood pressure; increased viscosity as in hyperglycaemia and polycythaemia; circulating emboli; pyaemia.

Results. Depends on site of thrombus. Coronary thrombosis (p. 14). Cerebral thrombosis (p. 179). Deep vein thrombosis (p. 31). Arterial thrombosis cuts off blood supply to tissues distal to blockage. Unless collateral supply adequate, affected tissues die: gangrene or infarct. Venous thrombosis less disastrous unless massive, or unless emboli occur.

Treatment. Complete rest. Anticoagulants to prevent extension of clot. Occasionally surgical removal of clot. Antibiotics.

Anticoagulant drugs

Heparin
An anticoagulant substance which occurs naturally in all tissues. Produced by mast cells which lie close alongside capillaries. Interferes with thrombin action on fibrinogen and prolongs clotting time. Has a strong electronegative charge, hence can be neutralized by substances with positive charge such as protamine.

Therapeutically heparin administered in thrombosis to prevent extension of clot. Intravenous injection has immediate anticoagulant effect: dosage 25–75 mg 6 hourly. Dose adjusted before each injection to maintain clotting time below 20 minutes. Careful observation necessary to detect capillary bleeding — petechiae, haematuria, tender gums. If these occur, give protamine sulphate 1 per cent intravenously. Dose: same number of mg as heparin given during last 6 hours.

Prothrombin inhibitors
Two groups of drugs have this effect, derivatives of

dicoumarol and inandione. Both groups interfere with liver's production of prothrombin and their effects can be reversed with vitamin K. Drugs given orally. Full effect not apparent for 24–48 hours. Dosage adjusted to keep prothrombin activity between 10 and 30 per cent. Daily estimates of prothrombin activity for first week of therapy, then weekly. Observations for haemorrhage as with heparin.

Preparations. Bishydroxycoumarin (dicoumarol) initial dose 200–400 mg, half this on second day, maintenance dose according to prothrombin activity. Warfarin (Coumadin) initial dose 30–50 mg, second day half this, subsequently according to prothrombin activity. Phenindione (Dindevan) initial dose 200–500 mg in divided doses 2 or 3 times first day, 50–150 mg second day, maintenance doses according to prothrombin activity.

Blood grouping and transfusion

ABO grouping

Erythrocytes classified into 4 types according to presence of certain protein substances which, under suitable conditions, cause them to clump together, i.e. to agglutinate. Substances are agglutinogens. 'A' type agglutinogen occurs in 'A' type cells, 'B' type agglutinogen occurs in 'B' type cells, both types of agglutinogens occur in 'AB' cells, type 'O' cells have no agglutinogens.

When erythrocytes come in contact with plasma antibodies called agglutinins — anti-A and anti-B, agglutination occurs.

Cross matching recipient and donor blood.

Sample of recipient's serum mixed with sample of donor's erythrocytes. If agglutination occurs, bloods are incompatible. Generally it is safe for recipient to receive blood of own group.

Universal donor

Group O cells contain no agglutinogens and are therefore unaffected by agglutinins that may be present in recipient's blood. Hence, in emergencies, it is safe for any person to receive group O blood.

Universal recipient

Group AB blood contains no agglutinins hence it is safe for persons of group AB to receive any blood.

Other causes of agglutination. RH Factor

About 85 per cent of people have this factor and are called Rh positives. The remainder do not have it and are called Rh negatives. If an Rh negative receives Rh positive erythrocytes, either by way of transfusion or because erythrocytes from an Rh positive fetus cross placental barrier, Rh negative person becomes sensitized and produces antibodies in a similar manner to the mechanism for production of antibodies to bacteria. If on a future occasion more blood of Rh positive type is received, or if another Rh positive foetus is conceived, the antibodies will cause agglutination of the Rh positive cells.

Several other proteins can have a similar effect, Duffy, Lutheran, Kell, Lewis, Kidd, MNS, P, Diego. Comparatively rare and only of importance if a person has ever had a previous blood transfusion. If this fact is known, cross matching with cells known to have these proteins is necessary to exclude possibility of incompatibility.

Transfusion reactions

Agglutination causes erythrocytes to clump together into small aggregates which lodge in capillaries. Soon after, the clumped erythrocytes break down and liberate large quantities of haemoglobin into blood stream. Of no consequence if amount is small but large quantities can pass from glomerular capillaries into the nephrons. One function of kidney is to reabsorb water from filtrate and this may be sufficient to concentrate urine beyond saturation point for haemoglobin. The haemoglobin will then precipitate and block the nephrons. If severe enough, acute renal failure results. Detected early by rigors, anxiety, apprehension, pain in back, chest or abdomen, passage of red, clear urine (not clouded as with passage of red cells in urine).

Treatment. (1) Stop transfusion at once; (2) give copious fluids; (3) render urine alkaline to raise saturation point for haemoglobin; (4) give diuretics.

Overtransfusion

Circulatory system overloaded with more blood than it normally contains.

Cause. Patient usually deeply shocked from haemorrhage. Blood given quickly to prevent death. As recovery from shock occurs and blood pressure rises to normal it is discovered that more blood than necessary has been transfused. Also in too rapid transfusion of whole blood in anaemia.

Signs and symptoms. Skin becomes tomato red. Blood pressure high. Pounding headache. Awareness of heartbeat. Oedema.

Treatment. Venesection.

Complications. Haemorrhage especially from wounds. Pulmonary oedema. Heart failure.

Erythroblastosis fetalis

Haemolytic condition of fetus due to passage of antibodies against Rh positive blood from mother to child. Mother is almost always Rh negative and has been sensitised against Rh positive blood by a previous pregnancy or by transfusion with Rh positive blood. If latter cause, tends to be severe. Occurs in 0·1–0·3 per cent of births. Each successive pregnancy with Rh positive child increases production of antibodies in mother's blood. First child usually normal, second child born jaundiced, third child severely affected or even stillborn.

Diagnosis. If mother known to be Rh negative, blood is tested for presence of antibodies.

Prophylaxis. Immunization of women at risk, using gammaglobulin containing high titre of anti-D.

Signs and symptoms. Child born anaemic and jaundiced; placenta enlarged; vernix caseosa, fatty substance covering child at birth, bright yellow; spleen enlarged.

Dangers. Free haemoglobin in blood stream quickly converted into bilirubin. Bilirubin excreted by liver as bile pigments but ability to do this is not fully matured in newborn, hence bilirubin accumulates. If level rises above 20 mg per cent, brain cells damaged permanently — kernicterus.

Treatment. Daily estimations of bilirubin necessary. If 20 mg per cent or more — exchange transfusion with Rh negative blood. Repeat if necessary.

Complications. Brain damage. Cirrhosis of liver.

2. The Respiratory System

Diseases of the respiratory system: sinusitis

Inflammation of mucous membrane lining nasal sinuses. Most commonly affected sinus — maxillary (antrum of Highmore); frontal and sphenoidal less commonly affected.

Acute

Cause. Secondary to viral infection. Occasionally streptococci, staphylococci, haemophilus.

Signs and symptoms. Pain in face below eyes, worse on bending forward; headache, particularly severe and persistent in sphenoidal sinusitis; general toxaemia varying from mild to severe.

Treatment. Antibiotics, sulphonamides, decongestants, antihistamines.

Chronic

Becoming rare because of effectiveness of chemotherapy.

Cause. Chronic thickening of mucous membrane, loss of cilia, blockage of hiatus.

Signs and symptoms. Chronic nasal discharge; 'post-nasal drip'; pain may be severe and persistent; chronic toxic absorption causing low level of general health, tendency to develop respiratory infections.

Treatment. Chemotherapy. Surgical provision of free drainage into nose.

Hay fever

Allergic rhinitis usually seasonal and accompanied by conjuctivitis.

Causes. Sensitivity to foreign protein, most commonly pollen from grasses, trees, flowers. Occasionally — fur, hair, feathers.

Signs and symptoms. Usually young adults; sometimes a history of asthma, urticaria or other allergic condition; sometimes family history; continuous watery discharge from nose; conjuctivitis and tears; headache and general depression; occasionally bronchitis and cough; simulates common cold but lasts longer.

Treatment. During attack: antihistamines — Benadryl, Anthisan etc; vasoconstrictors, nasal decongestants.

Preventive: Avoid contact if cause known. Discover causative agent with prick tests. Immunize with course of minute injections of causative agent.

Polypi

Tags and wormlike outgrowths of mucous membrane. May occur from any mucous surface. Often hereditary predisposition. Often multiple. Occasionally become malignant.

Signs and symptoms. In nose — nasal twang to voice; epistaxis; repeated respiratory infections.

Treatment. Removal. Wire snare tends to cause profuse bleeding. Cautery.

Enlarged adenoids

Adenoids — two collections of lymphoid tissue analogous with tonsils. They form a protective ring — Waldeyr's ring — round entrances to body. Together with deep and superficial cervical lymph nodes they protect against infection. Instrumental in establishment of immunity against bacteria hence their importance, especially in childhood, and surgeons' reluctance to remove them at an early age.

Gross enlargement blocks posterior nares and Eustachian tubes. Child is a mouth breather and is slightly deaf. Mouth breathing causes repeated respiratory infections; deafness, causes backwardness in school; blocked nose causes absorption of toxins. Combinations of these gives rise to typical appearance of pale unhealthy child with open mouth, runny nose, dark rings below eyes. Removal of adenoids brings about quick and dramatic improvement in such cases.

Acute streptococcal tonsillitis

Painful inflammation of tonsils with general toxaemia.

Signs and symptoms. Sore throat, pain, difficulty in swallowing. Tonsils swollen and inflamed. Follicles filled with pus which shows as white or yellow spots; pus can be expressed with swab. Deep and superficial cervical lymph nodes may be swollen or tender. General symptoms of toxaemia, may be severe — temperature 38–40°C, rapid pulse, headache, anorexia, diminished concentrated urine, malaise, mental depression.

Treatment. Rest in bed. Mouthwashes and gargles good psychologically. Prompt treatment with sulphonamides and/or penicillin because of danger of rheumatic diseases in particular and other possible complications in general. Diet soft and mushy until swallowing less painful. No particular restrictions.

Complications. Otitis media; mastoiditis; meningitis; encephalitis. Rheumatic group — nephritis, arthritis, chorea, any of the carditis group. (Rare with chemotherapy).

Acute tonsillitis pharyngitis, laryngitis, tracheitis

Often occur together with one part more severely affected. Inflammation of mucous lining.

Causes. Coincident with many infections — measles, whooping cough, diphtheria. Virus and bacterial infections of throat. Non-infectious causes — over-use of voice, gases, smoke.

Signs and symptoms. Sore throat; pain on swallowing; hoarseness or loss of voice; irritant unproductive cough usually worse at night; general symptoms not usually marked unless accompanying specific infectious diseases.

Treatment. Rest in bed while temperature raised; rest voice — provide pad and pencil or permit only whispering and only when essential; nurse in warm, moist atmosphere — steam kettle, or steam tent if severe; steam inhalations at frequent intervals; soothing linctuses if cough troublesome and unproductive; pastilles and lozenges to suck; chemotherapy if bacterial infection suspected.

Croup (laryngo-tracheo-bronchitis)

Inspiratory wheeze or crowing noise. A serious condition in babies and small children owing to narrow lumen of glottis and bronchioles. Inflammatory process may be sufficient to block them completely. Mucus becomes very thick and tenacious because of evaporation thus increasing danger of blockage.

Cause. Para-influenza or respiratory syncytial virus. A similar condition may arise in the course of other upper respiratory tract infections.

Signs and symptoms (other than of the underlying disease). *Stage 1*. Fever; hoarse voice; barking cough; inspiratory stridor. *Stage 2*. Continuous stridor; rib retraction on inspiration; accessory muscle brought into use during inspiration — sternomastoids, ala nasi; dyspnoea. *Stage 3*. Restlessness; anxiety (carbon dioxide retention, oxygen lack); pallor; sweating; rapid, shallow respirations; intermittent cyanosis. *Stage 4*. Increasing cyanosis becoming permanent.

Treatment. Barrier or isolation nursing; steam tent; constant reassurance; change bedclothes and nightgown frequently because steam makes them cold and uncomfortable; fluid intake maintained with encouragement and variety (intravenous fluids if necessary); antibiotics; observe closely for increasing obstruction; report at once if patient passing to lower stage; intensify observations and prepare for tracheotomy or intubation.

The following are not used: oxygen — it masks cyanosis and blockage can reach lethal stage without sufficient warning. Sedatives — mask restlessness and anxiety, child apparently sleeping peacefully but may be close to death. Atropine — makes sputum even more tenacious than it is already. (Oxygen and sedatives may be used *after* the decision to perform tracheotomy).

Complications. Glottal oedema; glottal spasm; atelectasis; pneumonia; lung abscess.

Tracheotomy (*Tracheostomy*)

Once the decision has been made to operate it is usually done promptly. Necessary instruments kept sterilized for immediate use.

Nurse's duties

Wrap child securely to prevent arm movement. Hold child's head firmly in straight line with body throughout operation — small movements of head cause great deviation of trachea. Concentrate on child — not on operation.

Local anaesthetic injected. Vertical incision, usually below cricoid cartilage. As soon as trachea opened dilators inserted and trachea sucked out. An outer tube, of suitable size, inserted and taped securely. An inner tube also inserted.

Care of patient

Nursed in steam tent and never left unattended. Steam keeps mucus fluid, easily sucked out. Often relief of cyanosis dramatic and child sleeps deeply. Observe respirations carefully — should be free and inaudible. Suck out immediately if 'bubbly'. Technique of sucking out — use sterile narrow gauge catheter, establish suction, pinch catheter, turn patient's head to one side, insert catheter gently, unpinch and withdraw catheter with a rotary action. (Wash catheter out by sucking sterile water or sterile bicarbonate of soda solution through it). Repeat with head turned to other side. (Turning head encourages catheter to enter opposite bronchus). Repeat until no evidence of mucus remaining. Do not poke catheter in and out. Remove inner tube at least daily and replace immediately with fresh sterile one, more often if evidence of mucus drying and scaling on it. Outer tube removed only by doctor. Petroleum jelly gauze keyhole dressing slipped between inner tube and skin, renewed daily or more often if soiled.

In some hospitals sterile sodium bicarbonate solution is instilled into tracheostomy with a sterile eye dropper. This liquefies mucus and humidifies inspired air. (It is claimed that sodium bicarbonate paralyses cilia and it is not allowed in many hospitals).

Removal of tracheotomy tube is usually possible 2–3 days later and stoma closes spontaneously without stitching. Cover with dressing to prevent 'fingering' and infection. If tube left longer than 3 days seal with sterile rubber cork for 3–4 hours before removal to reassure child that he can breathe normally.

Chronic bronchitis

Definition. Productive cough and mucoid sputum for 3 months or more in 2 successive years.

Causes. Cigarette smoking (in U.S.A. 75 per cent of cases smoke heavily). Other irritants — air pollutants e.g. sulphur dioxide.

Contributory factors and associated conditions. Acute

pneumonia, acute bronchitis, chronis sinusitis, congestion of the lungs, tuberculosis, pneumoconiosis.

Emphysema follows chronic bronchitis in a high proportion.

Pathology. Hyperplasia and hyperactivity of mucus secreting glands of bronchi and goblet cells of bronchial endothelium. Mucous membrane is roughened, thick, red, granular and may show loss of cilia and later metaplastic changes.

Signs and symptoms. Cough and sputum, usually history of smoking. Infective episodes with more copious yellow sputum Cough worse on waking and on exposure to irritants, e.g. dust, smoke, fumes. Dyspnoea not a major feature unless emphysema complicates the condition which it frequently does.

Course. Patient may continue coughing and spitting for years without further disability. Others progress through repeated acute episodes to obstructive pulmonary disease and emphysema, cor pulmonale.

Treatment. Must stop smoking. Antibiotics given during acute episodes. Bronchodilators and mucolytic agents, e.g. bromhexene helpful. Avoid inhalation of irritants.

Bronchiectasis

Dilatations along course of bronchi, replacement of their cartilage with fibrous tissue, destruction of mucous lining and loss of ciliated surface cells.

Cause. Increased tension on bronchial walls. Frequently follows atelectasis in which no air can enter collapsed section but the extra-bronchial pull during inspiration still occurs.

Signs and symptoms. Paroxysmal coughing with copious thick, offensive, purulent sputum. Haemoptysis — often streaking of sputum with blood — rarely frank haemoptysis. Generally — dyspnoea on exertion, readily contracts respiratory infections, pallor due to toxic absorption from lungs, clubbing of fingers common.

Diagnosis. Bronchogram shows dilatations.

Treatment. Aimed at keeping lungs drained of mucus and free from infection. Postural drainage 3 times daily especially first thing in morning; more frequently if necessary. Chemotherapy at once if infection occurs. Surgical resection if confined to one lobe or one lung. Stop smoking.

Complications. Sepsis; lung abscess; brain abscess; pneumonia; pleurisy; pericarditis; arthritis; cor pulmonale.

Asthma

A hyper-reactive response to inhalation of foreign protein — dusts, pollens, fur, feathers, smoke — in which spasm of the bronchioles occurs and lining mucous membrane becomes swollen and oedematous thus narrowing lumen of bronchioles to such an extent that free entry and exit of air into air sacs grossly impeded.

Signs and symptoms. Onset in childhood. Often a personal history of allergies — hay fever, skin reactions etc. Sometimes a similar family history. Sometimes a psychological factor precipitates attack — death of relative, anticipation of special event, e.g. special treat, visit of a favourite person, approaching examination. Sometimes attack initiated by infection. Often attacks diminish in number and intensity as child grows up. Occasionally progresses to chronic asthma.

During attack. Sudden onset, often at night; dyspnoea severe especially on expiration; audible wheezing; child sits upright or leaning forward with knees raised to obtain full benefit of abdominal pressure against diaphragm, head thrown back and accessory muscles brought into play. Often very frightened and this may be made worse by sudden concern of parents, visit from doctor and immediate transfer to hospital. Cyanosis denotes very severe attack.

Treatment. During attack. Beta-receptor agonist drugs cause relaxation of bronchial smooth muscle. Allows air to reach alveoli more readily thus improving gas exchange. Orciprenalin (Alupent) 0:5 to 1:0 mg i.m. or i.v., terbutaline sulphate (Bricanyl) 5–15 ml of elixir orally or 0:25 mg s.c.; ethylnoradrenaline (Bronkephrine) 2 mg/ml s.c. or i.m.

Aminophylline 250 mg/10 ml i.v. or 500 mg/2 ml i.m. or suppository 250 mg.

Direct inhalation of bronchodilators very effective especially if vaporized with pressure pump or venturi mask attached to Bird or Bennett respirator. Salbutamol (Ventolin); isoprenaline (Isuprel) terbutaline (Bricanyl).

Metered aerosol inhalers available and very effective. Oxygen may be given freely. Sedatives avoided if attacks moderate to severe or frequently repeated, steroids given, e.g. hydrocortisone 100 mg but a course of steroids or their use in every case is not recommended.

Between attacks: Metered aerosol inhalers of betameclasone (Becotide, Aldecin) stabilise cell membranes and reduce release of local histamines. Two puffs four times daily. Far lower systemic effects than oral steroid preparations. Sodium cromoglycate (Intal) by inhalation of ultrafine powder through special centrifuge device (Spinhaler). Very effective in reducing number of attacks and severity of attacks. Stabilises cells which liberate histamines, kinins, believed to initiate attacks.

Occasionally asthma presents in severe, life threatening form. Bronchospasm coupled with mucous membrane oedema and thick tenacious sputum may require tracheostomy, positive pressure ventilation with Bennett respirator, together with oxygen, humidification, suction and full drug utilisation, steroids i.v., aminophylline, beta adrenergic agonists.

Respiratory or intensive care unit with constant monitoring of respiratory volume and excursion, arterial blood gas analysis and control of fluid and electrolyte balance.

General treatment. Education of parents who are often over-solicitous and over-protective; encourage active participation in children's games especially in open air; avoid over-clothing of child. If allergic factors predominate — eliminate sources of dust, use rubber filled pillows and mattress, linoleum on floor, nylon or other synthetic fibres for clothing, check domestic pets and keep them out of bedroom especially.

A course of physiotherapy may help. Child taught exercises to be performed at home twice daily — to develop and encourage deep breathing.

Chronic asthma

Wheezing continues almost continuously with acute attacks occurring from time to time. Often hard to distinguish from chronic bronchitis. Child should be encouraged to continue going to school and, as far as possible, should not be treated as a chronic invalid. Exercises such as walking in fresh air at own pace encouraged. Sometimes onset of acute attack heralded by attack of hay fever and may be aborted with isoprenaline or aminophylline. Deep breathing exercises, especially those that encourage development of expiratory muscles should be carried out more frequently.

Emphysema

Definition. Condition of lung characterized by increase beyond the normal, in the size of air spaces distal to the terminal bronchioles, either from dilatation or from destruction of their walls. (Ciba Symposium 1959).

Causes. Smoking undoubtedly plays important part and 70 per cent of sufferers are smokers. Close association with chronic bronchitis. Factor contributing to chronic bronchitis also found in emphysema, e.g. cold damp climate, dusty working conditions, polluted urban environment.

Other causes of partial bronchial obstruction may lead to emphysema, e.g. bronchogenic carcinoma, pneumoconiosis, repeated attacks of pneumonia, long standing pulmonary tuberculosis.

Pathology. Chronic bronchiolitis, intraluminal granulation tissue, loss of alveolar elastic tissue, obliteration of alveolar walls, resulting in large inelastic air spaces, loss of capillaries. Fixation of alveoli in state of full expansion, inability to dilate further, so little air enters; inability to contract so little air leaves; result — alveolar stagnation and interference with gas exchange.

Signs and symptoms. Thorax fully expanded and fixed — 'barrel' chest; accessory muscles of respiration stand out — sterno-mastoids and scalenes; respirations gasping; dyspnoea especially on even slight exertion; cyanosis sometimes severe; cough usual — chronic bronchitis; round shoulders; neck veins prominent.

X-ray shows hyperinflated chest, flattened diaphragm, bullae. Vital capacity and forced expiratory volume in 1 second (FEV_1) reduced. Arterial oxygen partial pressure reduced while carbon dioxide pressure increased. In established cases respiratory acidosis is constant. Usually respiratory acidosis causes deeper, faster respirations — the normal respiratory control mechanism — but in emphysema this mechanism fails and rate and depth regulated by oxygen need. Hence if patient given oxygen at high rate apnoea occurs and patient may die from CO_2 retention.

Treatment. Entirely symptomatic. Treat respiratory infections promptly.

Lung abscess

Localised collection of pus within lung.

Cause. Always secondary to: (1) inspiration of infected material — tooth, pus from peritonsillar abscess, material from opposite lung; (2) suppuraton of pneumonic area; (3) extension of infection — liver abscess, subphrenic abscess, infected emboli.

Signs and symptoms. Pyrexia; rigors; sweating; dyspnoea; cough with foul sputum; pleuritic pain; clubbing of fingers which may develop very rapidly; leucocytosis; X-ray shows consolidated rounded mass, with fluid level in it.

Treatment. Antibiotics. Surgical drainage, lobectomy, pneumonectomy if no sign of resolution.

Complications. Pleurisy, with effusion; empyema. Gangrene of lung. Haemoptysis. Pericarditis. Brain abscess.

Pulmonary embolism

Blockage of pulmonary artery, or more commonly one of its branches, so that blood supply to part of lung is cut off.

Cause. Emboli passing through venous side of circulation and right side of heart. Sources — most commonly femoral thrombus, others — post-partum thrombi, post-surgical air emboli especially from prostate bed, malignant material from liver, mural clots from right atrium in atrial fibrillation, infarction material from right ventricle.

Signs and symptoms. Depends on extent of lung affected. Main pulmonary artery blocked — sudden substernal pain, rapid unconsciousness and death. One lung — sudden pain, dyspnoea, cyanosis, severe shock. Smaller area — dyspnoea, pleural pain, haemoptysis. X-ray may show dilation of pulmonary artery, elevation of diaphragm, opacity in lung, pleural effusion. Lung scan shows wedge-shaped area where blood fails to penetrate.

Treatment. Prevention of commonest source of emboli — leg exercises while in bed, early ambulation, eliminate anything constrictive around calf or thigh, remove knee pillows, elevate foot of bed and elevate legs while patient sitting out of bed. Pre-operative heparin. Calf stimulation during surgery. Inspect legs for pain and tenderness, discolouration, swelling.

If thrombosis suspected — bandage firmly with crepe bandage, cancel exercises, elevate leg on pillows, give anticoagulant for one week or longer if condition persists, to prevent extension of clot.

During attack — nurse in upright position; give oxygen; antibiotics to prevent infection of lung infarct; anticoagulants — heparin for 7–10 days, then warfarin for 6–12 weeks, analgesics.

Complications. Occurrence of further emboli. Death.

Pulmonary new growths

Most common form of cancer in males.

Types. 1. Squamous cell carcinoma 60 per cent (S.C.C.) (Epidermoid). Almost always associated with cigarette smoking. Usually arises in the hilar region. May produce obstructive signs early. Early spread to mediastinal glands.

2. Adenocarcinoma 15 per cent (Columnar cell carcinoma) (C.C.C.). Arise more commonly in periphery, sometimes associated with lung scars and chronic interstitial fibrosis, frequently spreads via bloodstream. Secondaries may give rise to initial symptoms.

3. Undifferentiated carcinomas (Anaplastic).
   (a) Large cell.
   (b) Small cell (oat cell carcinoma).
4. Large variety of rare tumours.
5. Metastatic.
(Many other classifications exist.)

Prognosis. Poor. Less than 5 per cent five year survival with any form of treatment.

Cause. Unknown but definite link with cigarette smoking.

Signs and symptoms. Insidious onset. Sometimes persistent cough with dyspnoea on exertion. Depends on site of growth — round bronchial roots, dyspnoea may be marked especially if atelectasis occurs; pleural surface — pain severe but little dyspnoea. Later — rapid loss of weight, toxaemia, pallor, weakness, oedema of thorax and face, hoarseness of voice if recurrent laryngeal nerve involved, X-ray may show growth but unilateral atelectasis more likely.

May present with unusual signs and symptoms, extreme muscle weakness, peripheral neuritis, rapid finger clubbing, raised serum calcium, flushing and burning from raised serum serotonin, low serum sodium.

Diagnosis. Sputum examined for malignant cells. Bronchoscopy and brush or forceps biopsy. Bronchial washings examined for malignant cells. Scalene lymph node biopsy. Needle biopsy of lung useful in peripheral lesions.

Treatment. Surgical removal — pneumonectomy usually but lobectomy possible with early diagnosis. If inoperable — some relief from pleuritic pain with deep X-ray therapy. Results with cytotoxic agents disappointing.

Pulmonary tuberculosis

Most common form of tuberculosis. Infectious disease spread by droplet infection from an existing case. Primary infection rarely serious and usually unnoticed. Tubercle bacilli treated like any other infecting organism — antibodies produced, but about 6 weeks after infection tissues become sensitized to tuberculoproteins. Clinical pulmonary tuberculosis arises after this incubation period, may be many years after, if organism not eradicated from the body and if contributory factors reduce effectiveness of body's defences. It is possible that some cases arise from re-infection.

Cause. Mycobacterium tuberculosae (tubercle bacillus, Tb).

Contributory factors

Incidence of tubercle bacillus so widespread that everybody would get tuberculosis if inhalation of organism was the only requirement. Organism alone is of low infectivity — takes advantage of reduced general level of health, hence factors which lower general health of equal importance — malnutrition, especially chronic shortage of proteins, poor housing conditions, overcrowding, lack of exercise, lack of fresh air, alcoholism, continued fatigue, existence of other infections and diseases.

Racial lack of resistance in peoples who have never contacted disease previously. Disease is not hereditary though reduced ability to build up immunity may be. Though there are many instances of several persons in one family with tuberculosis this is due to frequent exposure and likelihood of breadwinner being unable to provide adequately to stave off the other contributory factors.

The tubercle bacillus

Short rod which stains red with Gram's stain (Gram negative). Protected by outer fatty sheath which resists staining initially but protects stain from attempts to bleach it out with acids or alcohol (acid — alcohol fast, hence sometimes referred to as AAFB). Protective sheath also renders organism resistant to drying and cold, can survive for weeks in dust. Easily killed by heat — 60°C kills in 2 seconds. Grows slowly on culture medium 4 –6 weeks to produce visible colonies. Guinea pig peculiarly susceptible to infection, injection of suspected material in which no bacteria have been discovered by other means may cause death of guinea pig from generalised tuberculosis in 3–4 weeks.

Bovine strain can infect humans, usually by ingestion of infected milk. Bone and joint tuberculosis and cervical lymphadenitis results.

Pathology

Bacilli settle in wall of bronchiole or alveolus. Quickly surrounded by white cells especially giant monocytes. Outer layers proceed to fibrosis and later calcification in favourable cases. Inner parts soften to caseous material which may escape and set up fresh foci. Foci tend to run together causing cavitation. Areas around cavities infiltrated and oedematous.

Skin tests

Preparation, tuberculin, containing tuberculo-proteins used. Person primarily infected is sensitive to tuberculin. Tuberculin may be applied in several ways, most commonly intradermally. *Mantoux test* (most common test in Australia) — intradermal injection of tuberculin strength 1 in 1000; *Heaf test* (most common test in developing countries) — multiple puncture of epidermis with special 'gun' through a layer of filter paper soaked in tuberculin strength 1 in 1000 or 1 in 100; *Volmer test* — tuberculin jelly applied to skin and covered with adhesive; other tests less likely to give reliable results.

Site of test inspected after 24 hours. Positive reaction denoted by area covered with tiny vesicles surrounded by inflammation indicates sensitivity to tuberculin and immunity is presumed (but not proved). Violent or very extensive reactions may indicate active disease and X-ray is taken.

Prophylaxis

Active immunity conferred by injecting avirulent organisms. Practised in some countries since 1925. Organism used is usually BCG (bacille Calmette-Guerin) named after its discoverers — a naturally occurring strain isolated initially from a calf.

Signs and symptoms

Onset. Usually insidious with nothing definite until fairly advanced. Occasionally abrupt with haemoptysis or pleurisy or spontaneous pneumothorax, or pneumonic attack resembling influenza.

Cough. Persistent and worse on rising becoming gradually productive.

Sputum. Little at first — mucoid then muco-purulent.

Temperature. Slightly elevated in the evenings 37·5–38°C, slightly depressed in the mornings. Great care needed to establish this pattern otherwise it is easily missed.

Pulse. Slightly raised rate. Exercise tolerance test shows pulse slow to return to normal.

Respirations. Breathlessness on exertion.

Mental state. Malaise, disinterest in things previously found absorbing.

Nutritional state. Anorexia. Gradual loss of weight at first. May be extreme in advanced disease.

Others. Severe sweating while asleep. ESR raised — not diagnostic but a good indication of effectiveness of treatment.

Diagnosis

X-ray usually shows 'shadow'; may show cavitation. Sputum smears reveal tubercle bacillus — not always easy to find. Repeated morning specimens taken, occasionally fasting juice from stomach taken on waking. Culture to demonstrate absence of bacilli before discharge of patient.

Treatment

Rest in bed while febrile. Isolate while sputum positive. Antitubercular drugs (see below) hasten sputum conversaion and reduce isolation time. Previously, sanatorium regime — prolonged rest, fresh air, graduated exercises, collapse therapy effected many cures. Now modified because of effectiveness of drugs.

Anti-tubercular drugs. Streptomycin. Antibiotic with marked anti-tubercular activity. Must be given intramuscularly in doses not exceeding 1 g daily. Side effects — skin rashes, malaise, fever, eosinophilia; with prolonged administration — damage to 8th cranial nerve — vertigo, tinnitus, deafness, ataxia from which recovery may be slow or incomplete.

INAH (Iso-nicotinic acid hydrazide). Cheap easily produced chemical for oral administration. Dose 200–300 mg daily. Side effects — rare but incidence rises with increasing dosage — peripheral neuritis, insomnia, headache, constipation, dryness of mouth. High dosage in normal individuals may produce epileptiform fits hence administration to epileptics must be supervised with care. Most of side effects involving nerves can be controlled with coincident doses of pyridoxine (vitamin B6).

Rifampicin. Semisynthetic. Usually combined with INAH. Dose 600 mg daily. Well tolerated. May cause nausea, vomiting, diarrhoea.

Ethambutol. Dose 15 mg/kg/day orally in single dose often combined with streptomycin. Well tolerated. May cause retrobulbar neuritis.

PAS (para-amino salicylic acid). A white powder synthetically prepared. Irritant to gastric mucosa unless taken in enteric coated tablets. Dosage 10–15 g daily. Side effects — nausea, vomiting, diarrhoea which tend to disappear after few days administration. More serious but uncommon — kidney damage with albuminuria, haematuria; hepatitis; skin eruptions; agranulocytosis; goitre.

Cycloserine. An antibiotic extracted from *Streptomyces orchidaceus*. Good anti-tubercular activity when combined with one of the other drugs mentioned. Dosage 250 mg twice daily at 12 hourly intervals. Side effects — central nervous system depression — drowsiness, dizziness, mental confusion, convulsions. Incidence reduced if pyridoxine given at same time.

Pyrazinamide (pyrazomic acid amide). A synthetic white powder with high antitubercular activity but highly toxic. Used for short term therapy to cover surgery and only when close observation to detect early liver damage is possible. Dose not more than 35 mg per kg body weight and course not to exceed 6 weeks. Toxicity — liver damage which may be progressive and fatal after withdrawal of drug. Early symptoms — jaundice, raised SGOT. Also encourages uric acid retention and may bring on severe attack of gout.

Viomycin. An antibiotic produced by *streptomyces floridae*.

Complications

Spread of organism to other parts — larynx, pleura, pericardium. Blood borne to brain, meninges, kidneys, bones, joints; urinary spread from kidneys to ureters, bladder, testes; swallowed sputum to intestines — enteritis, peritonitis, ischio-rectal abscess.

Acute complications. Haemoptysis, spontaneous pneumothorax, pleural effusion.

Atelectasis

Alveoli completely empty of air, lung solid. Two varieties: (1) Congenital — air has failed to enter lung immediately after birth. (2) Acquired — blockage in bronchus, air distal to blockage absorbed. (Only acquired variety discussed here).

Cause. Blockage may be sudden — thick plug of mucus, inhaled foreign body, or it may develop slowly — gradual occlusion by new growth, pressure by enlarged gland.

Signs and symptoms. Depend on size of affected portion of lung and suddenness of blockage; large volume affected — dyspnoea, cyanosis, shock; small volume affected-breathlessness on exertion.

X-ray shows collapsed area. This may become infected causing pneumonia or lung abscess.

Treatment. Preventive — in any condition where mucus is thick and tenacious: (1) Give expectorants which liquefy mucus, avoid atropine which has reverse effect. (2) Give steam inhalations or nurse in steam tent. (3) Apply postural drainage with 'frappage' (rhythmic thumping with cupped hands over affected part). (4) Physiotherapy, deep breathing exercises, encourage vigorous coughing while supporting chest and any operation wounds. Analgesic drugs half hour before coughing help to make coughing more effective. (5) Encourage movement in bed and ambulate as soon as condition permits. (6) Repeated bronchial aspiration if tracheostomy present.

When atelectasis has occurred these measures must be intensified. Bronchoscopy and suction may help to clear obstruction but coughing still needed to re-expand airless volume.

Pleurisy

Inflammation of covering membranes of lung.

Causes. Spread of inflammation from neighbouring structures — tuberculosis, pneumonia, pericarditis, sub-phrenic abscess, carcinoma. Trauma to chest wall. Septicaemia. Direct viral involvement.

Types. 1. Acute, (a) with or (b) without fluid.
2. Chronic, (a) fibrous, (b) empyema.

Signs and symptoms

1a. Acute pleurisy with effusion. May follow dry pleurisy, abrupt cessation of pain as soon as layers of pleura are separated by fluid. If infected — rigors, fluctuation temperature. In tuberculous pleurisy with effusion — onset insidious, pain not severe. Signs and symptoms depend on (i) rate of development of fluid, (ii) amount of fluid. If large quantity develops rapidly — dyspnoea, cyanosis, displacement of mediastinal organs, deviation of trachea to opposite side, displacement of apex beat, pulse becomes rapid and may become irregular; dullness to percussion; X-ray shows dense shadow obliterating curve of diaphragm and obscuring lung.

1b. Acute dry pleurisy. Sudden onset with severe stabbing pain on deep breathing and coughing; cough dry and irritant; fever: 38–40°C; chest movements diminished; rate of respirations increased but not dyspnoeic; friction rub audible with stethoscope.

If pleurisy is diaphragmatic, pain is severe and is referred to neck or abdomen. Hiccoughs common.

Treatment

Acute dry. Nurse patient in upright position, treat underlying cause; give analgesics.

Treatment of effusion. Diagnostic aspiration. If infected, set up sensitivity tests and give appropriate antibiotic. Fluid aspirated only if (i) increasing in amount, (ii) dyspnoea marked, (iii) heart's action impeded, (iv) fluid persists and shows no reduction after 3–4 weeks.

Aspiration of chest (paracentesis thoracis). Preparation of patient. Reassure; explain in simple terms; warn against sudden movement or coughing without warning (morphine 15 mg may be given half hour before to reduce possibility of coughing). Position carefully so that patient is completely relaxed and well supported so that he can maintain position for as long as necessary; often position is sitting upright with arm raised above head and supported by nurse or leaning forward on pillow on table. *Nurse's duties during aspiration.* Mainly to look after patient; observe for reactions; encourage; support arm if procedure lengthy. *Possible reactions.* Sudden paroxysmal cough if local anaesthetic injected into lung. Pallor and fainting due to mediastinal shift if aspiration rapid or large amount removed: treatment — stop aspiration, reposition patient flat in bed with foot of bed raised. Spontaneous pneumothorax. Emphysema of chest wall. Slight haemoptysis if lung punctured.

Purulent pleurisy (Empyema)

Collection of pus in pleural cavity, usually walled off by adhesions and fibrin.

Causes. Usually pneumonia. Others — extension of disease, liver abscess, subphrenic abscess, peritonitis, tuberculosis; trauma — penetrating wounds of chest.

Signs and symptoms. Often masked by existing disease. May be pyrexia, rigors, sweating, pallor, dyspnoea if large quantity of pus, leucocytosis, anaemia.

Diagnosis. X-ray. Aspirate specimen.

Prognosis. Serious but very much improved with chemotherapy.

Treatment. Repeated aspirations. Instil antibiotic into space on alternate days after aspiration. Systemic antibiotics and/or sulphonamides. If cavity loculated by fibrous partitions it may be possible to break these down with injections of a fibrinolytic agent — streptokinase. This also helps to make the pus more liquid and easier to aspirate. Patient kept in bed if temperature raised but encourage to move about. Deep breathing exercises needed to help re-expansion of lung — blowing up balloons, blowing water from one bottle to another. *Surgical measures*. Rib resection, intercostal drain with suction through underwater seal; sometimes whole bag of pus can be excised completely.

Complications. Pericarditis, pneumothorax, lung abscess, bronchopleural fistula, nephritis.

Chronic pleurisy

Effusion may persist even after repeated aspirations without becoming purulent. Visceral pleura thickens and prevents re-expansion of lung. Chest wall becomes sunken and deformed. Scoliosis occurs — curvature of spine towards affected side.

Pneumothorax

Air in pleural cavity.

Types. *1. Artificial*. Air deliberately introduced via needle inserted between ribs. Formerly most common form of treatment for pulmonory tuberculosis.

2. Spontaneous. Break occurs in visceral pleura and air passes from lung into pleural space. Most common cause — tuberculosis. Others — cancer, emphysema. Occasionally idiopathic.

3. Tension. Special form of spontaneous pneumothorax in which valve-like action at break in visceral pleura prevents return of air into lung. Air enters pleural space during inspiration and fails to return during expiration. This is helped by natural tendency of lung to collapse so maintaining negative pressure within pleural space. If unrelieved, pump like action of respirations causes complete deflation of lung, compression of mediastinum which starts to compress opposite lung.

4. Traumatic. (Sucking wound of chest). Penetration of chest wall with or without fractured rib.

Signs and symptoms. None in spontaneous pneumothorax unless severe, and tension develops, then:– sudden onset of severe dyspnoea, pain, shock, pallor becoming cyanosis; mediastinum pushed to opposite side displacing apex beat; trachea displaced to unaffected side when head held in alignment with trunk. Percussion of affected side produces drum-like note, of unaffected side-dull note. No breath sounds heard on affected side. X-ray shows edge of collapsed lung against mediastinum.

Treatment. None in lesser degrees without mediastinal compression — air will reabsorb within 2–3 weeks.

In tension pheumothorax — puncture chest wall with wide bore plastic catheter and let air out. Connect to underwater seal bottle. Leak seals itself within 3–4 days and tube removed. Patient needs constant reassurance in first instance.

In traumatic pneumothorax — as first aid measure puncture in chest wall should be sealed as effectively as possible — pressure dressing or hand held firmly over layer of clean paper. Surgical treatment — suture wound, insert drainage tube at another point, connect to underwater seal drainage bottle. Removal possible after 2–4 days. Provide antibiotic cover.

Lobar pneumonia (Pneumococcal pneumonia)

An acute specific infectious disease of lungs.

Cause. Gram positive diplococcus — pneumococcus.

Aetiology. Occurs most commonly in children but no age group immune. Males more susceptible than females. Higher incidence in winter and spring. Often secondary infection superimposed. Spread by droplet infection hence epidemics occur in crowded conditions.

Pathology. One or more lobes affected in one lung; sometimes both lungs affected (double pneumonia). Capillaries engorged; alveoli fill with fibrin and blood cells; volume of lung consolidated. Later the blood cells are phagocytized, enzymes liquefy alveolar contents which are coughed up as 'rusty' sputum. Pleurisy invariable over affected parts.

Signs and symptoms. Abrupt onset with rigor in adults, convulsions in children. Temperature rises quickly to 39–40°C and remains elevated. Pleuritic pain often severe especially on deep breathing and coughing. Short dry cough. Respirations rapid and shallow, inspiration ends with a grunt of pain. Ala nasi muscles dilate with inspiration. Sputum scanty and tenacious at first, becomes more copious and rusty brown with blood cells later. Pulse full and bounding. Urine diminished and concentrated. Headache severe and persistent. Occasionally delirium. Herpes labialis common. Leucocytosis.

Course. All symptoms greatly relieved by chemotherapy. Untreated case temperature remains elevated for 7–10 days and falls dramatically by crisis. Patient becomes extremely toxic before crisis. Afterwards patient falls into deep, long sleep. Convalescence rapid.

Treatment. Nurse in upright position in warm but well ventilated room. Steam inhalations or steam tent in severe cases. Diet light and easily digestible. Copious fluids. Insomnia sometimes troublesome but controlled with sedatives. Morphia avoided because it depresses respirations and cough. As soon as sputum becomes free, postural drainage and breathing exercises started. Penicillin by injection initially 1−2 million units 6 hourly.

Prognosis. Excellent in 90 per cent of cases. Poor under 2 years of age or over 60. Poor risks: alcoholics, malnourished or obese patients.

Complications. Pleural effusion. Empyema. Myocarditis and heart failure. Meningitis. Arthritis. Recurrence. Severe toxaemia.

Bronchopneumonia

Not a specific infectious disease. Primarily a bronchiolitis. Patchy, widespread inflammation which may involve alveoli.

Causes. Pneumococci, staphylococci, streptococci, viruses, e.g. of measles, and influenza often a combination of haemophilus influenzae and *Strep. pneumoniae*. A serious condition in infants because of small size of bronchioles. Entry of bacteria may be due to inhalation of infected material — blood, pus, vomit. More common in patients after tracheotomy due to loss of cleansing action of nose. May spread from potentially infected conditions of lungs — bronchiectasis, lung abscess.

Signs and symptoms. Slight indisposition at first then pyrexia, cough, pain in chest, rapid respirations, tachycardia, cyanosis. X-ray — scattered shadowing throughout lung fields.

Treatment. Antibiotic to cover haemophilus — ampicillin, cotrimoxazole, tetracycline.

Other causes of pneumonia. Many bacteria responsible for forms of pneumonia neither truly lobar or bronchial. Some forms rapidly progressive, often fatal. Streptococcal often secondary to viral disease, e.g. influenza. Responds to penicillin.

Staphylococcal may follow influenza or occur in sickly children, premature infants, complicating other diseases in which cortico-steroids in use. Essential to establish antibiotic sensitivities as rapidly as possible. Cephalosporins, methicillin, ampicillin used initially.

Haemophilus, klebsiella, pseudomonas, proteus, isolated in individual cases under special circumstance. In each case appropriate treatment determined by early identification and sensitivity reactions.

Psittacosis (Ornithosis)

An acute infection of lungs resembling influenza.

Cause. Chlamidia present in faeces of birds. Caged birds spread disease to man — inhalation of dry, dusty droppings when cleaning cage.

Signs and symptoms. Malaise, fever, headache, generalised aching of limbs and joints, cough with little sputum. X-ray shows consolidation similar to lobar pneumonia.

Treatment. Chloramphenicol, tetracycline. Otherwise as for pneumonia.

Prognosis. High mortality. Importation of parrots and budgerigars from some parts of the world strictly controlled.

Sarcoidosis

Granulomatous condition of unknown aetiology, possibly viral, in which any tissues but notably lungs, may be infiltrated with lesions.

Signs and symptoms. May be symptom free even though X-ray shows gross changes. Occasonally cough, dyspnoea, weight loss. Granulomatous nodules may occur in skin, bones, joints, eyes, muscles, myocardium, lymph nodes.

Diagnosis. Kveim test — injection of antigenic material recovered from sarcoid nodules injected intradermally causes local reaction. Many false positives. Biopsy of skin or node most reliable, also needle biopsy of liver or lung. X-ray usually reveals dense bilateral hilar densities (Potato nodes). Lungs show 'snow-storm' effect.

Treatment. Nil specific Corticosteroids may speed up clearing on X-ray but not recommended unless symptoms marked.

Prognosis. Excellent. 95 per cent recover fully.

Pneumoconiosis (Industrial disease)

Inflammatory reaction and fibrosis of lungs following chronic inhalation of irritant dusts. May cause respiratory insufficiency. Often associated with emphysema. May progress to cor pulmonale.

Subdivisions

Silicosis from stone dust — stone masons, miners. Asbestosis — any form of handling asbestos from mining to manufacturing, e.g. brake linings. Anthracosis from mining anthracite coal. Siderosis — iron oxides from iron ore, electric arc welding.

Signs and symptoms. Gradual onset of increasing dyspnoea, cough, sputum. Frequent bronchitis attacks, haemoptysis may be severe. X-ray evenly scattered small opacities, hilar node enlargement. Fine linear markings of fibrosis.

Treatment. Nil specific. Remove from environment of causative agent. Encourage postural drainage. Treat infections early and vigorously.

Prognosis. Gradual deterioration. Eventual right sided heart failure. Carcinoma common termination in asbestosis. Tuberculosis may complicate silicosis.

Respiratory failure

Failure to effect gaseous exchange. May ensue from many causes, e.g. (1) obstruction — epiglottitis, carcinoma, inhaled foreign body, asthma, brochiolitis, emphysema. (2) fluid — drowning, pulmonary oedema, blood, pneumonia, pus. (3) restriction of respiratory movement or of lungs, obesity, abdominal distension, pleural effusion, pneumothorax, flair chest, atelectasis. (4) interference with innervation — poliomyelitis, myasthenia gravis, some drugs. (5) interference with blood flow to and from alveoli — pulmonary embolism, pulmonary hypertension, right ventricular failure.

Signs and symptoms. Of underlying disease plus restlessness, confusion, reduced BP, pallor or cyanosis, air hunger. CO_2 retention causes acidosis in acute respiratory failure but bicarbonate retention corrects this in chronic failure.

Diagnosis. Arterial blood gas measurement shows CO_2 partial pressure ($PaCO_2$) raised above 50 mmHg. Blood pH low in acute failure (respiratory acidosis). Normal in chronic failure but bicarbonate level raised. Low vital capacity.

Treatment. Best in intensive care unit where emergency facilities for intubation, tracheostomy, constant monitoring and specialist staff constantly in attendance.

Oxygen sufficient to keep PaO_2 between 50 and 60 mmHg. (Care needed in chronic failure in which respiratory centre operates on PaO_2 and not $PaCO_2$).

Drugs include those necessary to alleviate underlying condition — antibiotics, bronchodilators, humidifiers, expectorants, and those to correct acid/base balance.

Physiotherapy — should be instituted at earliest possible time. Patient cooperates if possible in active respiratory exercises, controlled coughing but passive postural drainage and thumping where patient unable to cooperate.

If necessary, respiration assisted or taken over by machine. Assistance machines (e.g. Bird), can be set to trigger by patients own inspiratory effort. Control machines (e.g. Bennet), can be set to deliver at predetermined rate, flow and O_2 concentration.

Monitoring of rate, peak pressure, tidal volume, PaO_2, $PaCO_2$, essential.

3. The Digestive System

The mouth

Oral cleanliness an important nursing duty. Infection occurs quickly in very ill patients. Can spread to (1) salivary glands; (2) middle ear; (3) digestive tract; (4) respiratory tract.

Patients who need special oral care. Those with any febrile condition; respiratory disease; unconscious or heavily sedated patients; those on fluid diet; those receiving atropine in any form; those with blood in mouth for any reason — dental extraction, tonsillectomy, haemoptysis, etc; those with conditions necessitating mouth breathing; tracheotomy.

Prevention of infection

Frequent washing with antiseptic lotions — glycerine of thymol, hydrogen peroxide, Milton; removal and thorough cleansing of dentures; use of toothbrush after eating but especially at night; chewing gum; application of emollient cream to lips — lanoline, petroleum jelly, zinc oxide, peppermint cream.

Diseases of the mouth: stomatitis

Inflammation of mouth.

Types

1. Catarrhal. Mucous membrane red, swollen and dry; gums sore and painful on chewing. Treatment as above. Treat underlying cause.

2. Aphthous. Crops of small ulcers appear on gums, cheeks and borders on tongue. Occurs commonly in debilitated children.

3. Thrush. Fungus with infection *Monilia albicans*. Most common in ill babies who are bottle fed. Also occurs when normal flora disturbed by powerful antibiotics. Monilia normally present in mouth, vagina, and on skin. Multiply when other commensals destroyed. Form greyish white membrane. Can spread rapidly to bronchi causing serious complication in babies and elderly sick. *Prevention*. Scrupulous cleanliness of feeding bottles, teats etc. *Treatment*. Nystatin (Mycostatin) 1 ml oral suspension dropped into mouth 4 times daily. Absorbed and acts systemically. No need to swab lesions individually.

4. Cancrum oris. Serious form of infection occurring in debilitated persons especially undernourished children with infectious diseases e.g. measles. Ulceration of inner surface of cheek, spreads and can erode through cheek. Frequently fatal but recovery possible with early diagnosis and penicillin.

5. Vincent's angina. An infectious stomatitis caused by a spirochaete and a bacillus occurring together. Often found in mouth without evidence of disease. May cause greyish membrane on tonsils resembling diphtheria. Other symptoms — sore tender gums, foul breath, occasionally general symptoms — malaise, slight temperature, enlarged cervical nodes. *Treatment*. Penicillin systemically; strict oral hygiene; destroy toothbrush when cured.

6. Drug stomatitis. May follow use of mercury, bismuth and other heavy metals.

7. Agranulocytosis. (p. 39). Often revealed early by ulceration of mouth or pharynx.

Diseases of salivary glands: mumps (epidemic parotitis)

Acute specific infection of salivary glands.

Cause. Virus. Spread by droplets.

Incubation period. 14–21 days.

Signs and symptoms. Swelling and tenderness of one parotid gland with the other affected commonly 2–5 days later. Submaxillary glands usually affected also. Sublingual glands rarely. Pain on opening mouth, on chewing and swallowing. Acid substances cause severe discomfort. Mouth dry. General symptoms — slight pyrexia.

Course. Glands swell to maximum in 3–4 days and subside in 7–10 days.

Complications. Rare. Orchitis (occasionally atrophy of testis and sterility). Oophoritis; encephalitis; pancreatitis; mastitis.

Treatment. Nil specific. Aspirin or other analgesic ½–1 hour before meals. Rest in bed while pyrexial. Mumps gamma globulin or mumps convalescent serum may reduce incidence of orchitis. *Treatment of complications*. Orchitis — elevate scrotum on elastoplast bridge between thighs. Codeine or morphine may be required for pain, or it may be controlled by injecting spermatic cord with procaine — 10 ml of 1 per cent solution. Hydrocortisone 100 mg i.v. and 20 mg orally for 3–5 days reduces inflammation. Encephalitis — lumbar puncture if headache severe. Hydrocortisone.

Prevention. Live attenuated mumps virus 0·5 ml at age 12 months.

Suppurative parotitis

Spread of infection from a 'dirty' mouth. Almost always preventable by nursing skill. Occurs most commonly in old persons nursed at home.

Signs and symptoms. Parotid gland (usually one only) swollen, painful, hot and tender to touch. Temperature elevated. Pus may be seen coming from Stenson's duct. Mouth dry. Tongue coated. Breath foul.

Treatment. Antibiotics. May be necessary to incise and drain.

Salivary calculi

Develop slowly. Most commonly obstruct Wharton's duct.

Signs and symptoms. Painful swelling of gland due to collection of saliva. May swell visibly before meal or when acid placed on tongue (vinegar).

Treatment. Dilation of duct and surgical removal of calculus.

Oral cancer

5 per cent of all cancers. Usually squamous cells, less commonly basal cell, rarely melanoma. May occur on any surface, cheeks, gums, tonsils, palate. Often preceded by leukoplakia (white, thickened, mucous membrane). Increased in smokers.

Signs and symptoms. Ulcer, usually painless at first, which fails to heal. Rolled, raised edge, hard indurated base. Excessive salivation. Adenitis — submaxillary and cervical.

Diagnosis. Cytology. Biopsy.

Treatment. Surgical excision. Radiation.

Prognosis. Depends on stage at which diagnosis made and extent of surgery.

Stage 1 — local ulcer without metastasis very good.

Stage 2 — ulcer with local node involvement 30 per cent 5 year survival.

Stages 3 and 4 — local and distant spread very poor.

The oesophagus: diseases of the oesophagus

Oesophagitis

Inflammation of oesophagus.

Causes. 1. Extension of inflammation from pharynx and larynx.

2. Swallowed irritants — corrosives, acids, alkalies, boiling water.

3. Regurgitation of acid contents of stomach.

4. Cancer.

Signs and symptoms. Pain on swallowing. Heartburn.

Treatment. Semisolid foods. Milk mixtures. Treat underlying cause.

Achalasia

Food fails to pass normally into stomach, though no obvious obstruction. Associated with loss of ganglion cells within muscle layers of at least some areas of affected oesophagus.

Dilatation and hypertrophy of lower end of oesophagus.

Signs and symptoms. Patient complains that 'food sticks'. Discomfort and feeling of fullness after eating. Not painful. Vomiting may occur ½ – 1 hour after meals and vomitus consists of recently eaten food and saliva.

Diagnosis. Confirmed by barium meal, shows dilated oesophagus.

Treatment. Teach patient to pass dilator — Hirst's mercury tube — rubber tube about ½ – ¾ in. thick weighted with mercury. In lesser degrees, relaxation of sphincter may be achieved by deep breathing, stretching or active exercise. Patient should avoid: extremely hot or cold drinks, 'fizzy' drinks, emotional upset.

Occasionally surgery is necessary — operation similar to Ramstedt's. (Muscle layer from 5 cm above sphincter to 5 cm below split longitudinally but mucous membrane left intact.)

Hiatus hernia

Definition. Herniation of portion of stomach into chest through oesophageal hiatus of diaphragm.

Types. (1) Sliding — most common. Abdominal part of oesophagus and portion of stomach slides above diaphragm.

(2) Para-oesophageal or rolling. Portion of stomach passes through hiatus and lies alongside oesophagus.

Signs and symptoms. Oesophagitis due to regurgitated gastric contents, made worse by stooping or when lying flat hence more severe at night. Restrosternal pain. Anaemia, belching, vomiting.

Diagnosis. Barium meal. Film taken when patient in Trendelenburg position shows kinking of the oesophagus at its lower end.

Treatment. Reduce reflux of gastric acid and neutralise effect on oesaphageal mucosa. Avoid large meals, keep meals as dry as possible, avoid drinks immediately after meals. Avoid bending. Elevate head of bed 10 to 15 cm. Avoid tight belt or other constriction round middle. Keep weight at optimum. Use antacids and alginic acid after meals.

Surgery avoided except in severe disabling cases or when fibrotic scarring interferes with swallowing.

Benign stricture

Contraction of scar tissue following swallowing of corrosives, foreign bodies, inflammatory conditions, peptic oesophagitis.

Signs and symptoms. Gradually increasing difficulty in swallowing until only liquids will pass. Patient complains of food 'sticking' and can often accurately indicate level of stricture.

Treatment. Dilatation with bougies. Gastrostomy may be needed temporarily to prevent extreme wasting. If dilatation impossible — resection of strictured portion and oesophago-gastrostomy.

Cancer of oesophagus

Signs and symptoms. Dysphagia rapidly progressing to inability to swallow anything except fluids. Emaciation rapid and extreme. Early discomfort progressing to constant pain at level of obstruction — sometimes experienced in back. Substernal pain after hot drink.

Diagnosis. Barium meal shows level of blockage. Oesophagoscopy and biopsy confirms diagnosis.

Treatment. Surgical — excision with oesophagoplasty. Palliative — intubation or gastrostomy to prevent starvation. Deep radiation therapy occasionally employed to prolong life.

The stomach

Dyspepsia

A common syndrome indicating faulty digestion which may or may not be indicative of serious disease.

Signs and symptoms. Epigastric discomfort after meals; feeling of fullness; heartburn; flatulence; nausea; occasional vomiting; furred tongue; constipation.

Vomiting

Regurgitation of contents of stomach, and sometimes of intestines.

Types and causes. 1. Reflex via glossopharyngeal nerve following stimulation of fauces, tonsils, pharynx, back of tongue. Usually mechanical — irritation by food, tablet, fishbone lodged in pharynx.

2. Reflex via vagus nerve following irritation of lining of stomach or intestine or stretching of intestinal wall. Disease processes — gastritis, ulcer, cancer, obstruction, paralytic ileus. Drug irritation — salt water, zinc sulphate, mustard.

3. Direct stimulation of vomiting centre in medulla oblongata. Mechanical — intracranial pressure. Psychological — unpleasant smells, sights etc. Neurological — Meniere's disease, travel sickness. Toxic — apomorphine, tobacco, alcohol, ipecacuanha. Toxaemic — uraemia, ketosis, pregnancy.

Other causes — pain, e.g. testicular trauma, stretching of tendons etc.

Observations of significance. (Nurse often only witness and valuable clues to cause may depend on her.) Onset — whether accompanied by nausea; any relation to food; to drugs recently administered. Whether preceded by salivation, or pallor. Did patient retch or was it effortless? Did it gush out in large quantity; was it repeated small quantities; was the patient relieved by vomiting or did nausea persist afterwards; what was the nature of the vomitus — any food in it, if so was it eaten recently; any particular odour; did it contain: tablets; blood; bile; faecal material?

Treatment. Support abdomen and forehead during attack. Remove soiled garments and bedclothes as soon as possible as smell may initiate further vomiting. Wash mouth, dentures, hands. If repeated — withhold food and drink — especially if surgery may be needed. Depending on cause it may be necessary to pass Ryle's tube and keep stomach empty. Nausea without vomiting sometimes controlled with chlorpromazine orally 10–50 *mg* 4–6 hourly.

Hiccough

Usually transient and of no significance. Persistent hiccough may be symptomatic of serious disease — peritonitis, subphrenic abscess, intestinal obstruction, paralytic ileus, cerebral tumour, uraemia, meningitis, diaphragmatic pleurisy.

Treatment. Progress from simple 'home' remedies to drugs. Holding breath, rebreathe from paper bag 3–4 minutes, drink glass of water without taking a breath. Inhale 5 per cent carbon dioxide; local anaesthetic to nasal mucous membrane (cocaine ½ per cent), atropine 0·3–0·6 mg subcutaneously, amyl nitrite ampoule broken and vapour inhaled, chlorpromazine 10–50 mg orally or intramuscularly, general anaesthetic.

Diseases of the stomach: Acute gastritis

Common condition due to inflammation of gastric mucosa.

Causes. Mechanical irritation — skins, pips, bones etc. Chemical irritation — alcohol, unfamiliar foods. Bacterial toxins, especially staphylococcal, that have accumulated in contaminated foods — pies, custards etc. Accompanying other conditions — diphtheria, measles, viral infections. Allergic response to some foods — shellfish, strawberries.

Signs and symptoms. Anorexia; fullness; nausea; vomiting; haematemesis; epigastric pain and tenderness; colic; diarrhoea. Dehydration and loss of electrolytes may be severe.

Treatment. Nothing by mouth until nausea, vomiting and pain cease, then progress, as tolerated without resumption of symptoms, through water, milk and water, whole milk, semisolid bland foods, solids to normal diet. If dehydration present, maintain adequate fluids intravenously. Electrolyte imbalance checked and corrected. If definite organism isolated in faeces — antibiotic or sulphonamide to which it is sensitive. Rest in bed while pyrexial.

Chronic gastritis

Trophic changes in stomach lining sometimes secondary to other conditions — ulcer, cancer, chronic irritation, deficiency of iron, but frequently of unknown origin.

Signs and symptoms. Anorexia; fullness; nausea; vomiting; haematemesis; occasionally, absence of hydrochloric acid.

Treatment. Treat basic cause if known. Others — often unsatisfactory; ulcer regime may help.

Peptic ulceration

Ulceration of those portions of digestive tract which may come in contact with gastric secretions. May be acute or chronic. About 10 per cent of gastric ulcers become malignant. Duodenal ulcer never becomes malignant.

Types. 1. Duodenal ulcer — 5 times more common than gastric ulcer.

2. Gastric ulcer.

3. Postoperative stomal (jejunal) ulcer.

Duodenal ulcer

Site. Almost all occur in the duodenal cap within 5 cm of the pyloric sphincter.

Signs and symptoms. Pain described as gnawing or burning; comes on 45–60 minutes after eating a meal; in epigastrium near xiphoid process; occasionally referred to back or right shoulder; pain relieved by vomiting or by taking milk, alkalis or food; pain often worse at night soon after falling asleep. Tenderness on palpation usually present.

Tests show hypochromic anaemia; occult blood in faeces; hyperacidity and increased secretion of gastric juice. X-ray may show ulcer crater but it may be difficult to demonstrate in old cases with much scarring. Other X-ray findings include increased peristalsis of stomach and duodenum and spasm of the pyloric sphincter. Duodenoscopy may reveal ulcer.

Treatment. Rest from work 2–3 weeks. Stop smoking. No

alcohol. Rest as much as possible but no need to confine to bed.

Diet. Full nutritional diet taken in small meals at 2 hourly intervals.

Antacids. Many antacids available and most are effective if taken regularly and in sufficient amount. During acute phase — every hour (during night as well in severe cases). As pain diminishes — every 2 hours. Aluminium hydroxide, 1–2 teaspoons or tablets, tablets should be chewed slowly and thoroughly. Magnesium trisilicate — same. (Aluminium compounds may cause constipation and are often combined with magnesium compounds which cause diarrhoea, the 2 substances off-setting each other). Others frequently used — calcium carbonate, bismuth subcarbonate, magnesium oxide.

Histamine H2 receptor antagonists. Cimetidine (Tagemet). Supresses acid secretion.

Oral administration 200 mg t.i.d., pc, and 400 mg nocte for one month brings about rapid elimination of symptoms. Ulcers frequently heal completely.

Relapse common but less likely with maintenance dosage of 400 mg nocte.

Newer H2 receptor antagonists which show great promise are ranitidine and tiotidine.

Mucosal barriers. Liquorice derivatives such as carbenoxolone (Biogastrone. Duogastrone) strengthen existing mucosal defences, perhaps by stimulating mucus secretion.

Duogastrone taken orally before meals, slow release capsules especially for duodenal ulceration.

Good healing claimed. May cause fluid and sodium retention and potassium depletion. Occasionally hypertension occurs and must be watched for.

Colloidal Bismuth salts. Tri-potassium dicitrato-bismuthate (De-Nol) promotes rapid healing of peptic ulcers.

General advice. Before releasing patient for self care he should be educated as to nature of disease. Points to stress — recurrent nature of condition under unfavourable circumstances (irregularity of meals, mental stress, excessive use of alcohol and tobacco, injudicious choice of foods); severe nature of possible complications; need to include a variety of permitted foods in diet; need for adequate rest each day, at least one day a week away from work.

Complications

(1) Haemorrhage; (2) Perforation; (3) Penetration; (4) Obstruction.

Haemorrhage. Often chronic small or continuous haemorrhage with consequent depletion of body iron and hypochromic anaemia. Due to capillary bleeding from granulating surface of healing ulcer. Sometimes massive, due to erosion of blood vessel with sudden onset of: weakness; sweating; pallor; rapid pulse; low blood pressure; diarrhoea with melaena; occasionally haematemesis. *Treatment*. Put to bed at once; keep warm without overheating; sedate but avoid morphia because it may cause vomiting and intensify shock; take blood sample for grouping and cross-matching; prepare for immediate setting up of intravenous drip (using saline until blood is ready); observe vital signs ½–1 hourly; pulse, blood pressure, temperature, respirations and record progress.

Patient probably nauseated and anorexic for first 24 hours but if not, some doctors like to start oral feeding — milk 50–100 ml hourly alternating with antacids. Meulengracht diet may be used i.e. full diet in puree form without irritant substances.

Perforation. Erosion through all layers of intestinal wall with spilling of contents into peritoneal cavity. Surgical emergency which needs immediate repair; usually simple closure, more extensive surgery not performed at this time because of patient's poor condition.

Signs and symptoms. Sudden onset of severe abdominal pain radiating to tip of right shoulder. Pain tends to lessen for a few hours and then returns as peritonitis develops with board-like rigidity of abdominal muscles, fever, rebound tenderness, tachycardia, absence of bowel sounds.

Treatment. Immediate surgical closure.

Penetration. Ulcer erodes through wall into adjacent organs to which duodenum adherent without spilling contents into peritoneal space. Occurs only in long standing cases.

Signs and symptoms. Intensification of symptoms with no relief from pain by taking antacids, food or by vomiting. Pain made worse by standing upright and stretching; relieved by leaning forward. Pancreas most commonly affected; may cause pan-

creatitis. Other organs — liver, gall bladder, bile ducts.
Treatment. Surgical.

Obstruction. May be due to local oedema and spasm during active phase of ulcer, or to contraction of scar tissue following healing. Former responds to ulcer treatment. Latter may need surgery.

Signs and symptoms. Of chronic type — gastric fullness and heaviness; vomiting of large quantity of fluid containing food eaten previous day. Gastric aspiration first thing in morning dilation and increased peristalsis.

Treatment. Partial gastrectomy and vagotomy.

Gastric ulcer

Ulceration of gastric mucous membrane associated with increased acidity of gastric juice and decreased tissue resistance.

Site. 85 per cent occur on or near lesser curvature of stomach and ⅔ of these within 7·5 cm of pyloric sphincter.

Occurrence. Men more than women (3:1) usually over 40 years. Often history of irregular meals and mental tension.

Signs and symptoms. Pain in epigastrium occurring 20–60 minutes after eating; tenderness on palpation; nausea and vomiting; appetite good but patient dreads eating; weight loss; anaemia; haematemesis.

Diagnosis. Confirmed by test meal which shows increased acid and free acid after injection of histamine. Gastroscopy — ulcer may be visualized. Barium meal may show ulcer crater and increased motility of stomach.

Treatment. As for duodenal ulcer. About 10 per cent of gastric ulcers progress to malignancy. If patient does not respond to treatment within 4–6 weeks some doctors recommend exploratory laparotomy followed by gastrectomy if necessary.

Evidence of more rapid healing with carbenoxolone (Biogastrone), liquorice derivative, dose 100 mg tid. Possible side effects — potassium depletion, renal failure, hypertension.

Zollinger-Ellinson syndrome

Excessive production of gastrin, often from pancreatic tumour, causes gastric hypersecretion. Peptic ulceration severe, multiple, resists treatment. Complications common.

Diagnosis. Serum gastrin levels greater than 300 pg/ml.

Treatment. Location and removal of tumour if possible. Frequently impossible however as tumour may be multiple and microscopic. Subtotal gastrectomy removes source of acid. Cimetidine (Tagemet) 200 mg t.i.d., p.c., 400 mg n.

Complications

Haemorrhage (haematemesis). Perforation. Obstruction (hour-glass stomach or pyloric stenosis). Malignancy.

Haematemesis. Vomiting of blood. May be 'true' — bleeding originating in stomach or oesophagus, or 'false' — regurgitation of swallowed blood from epistaxsis, haemoptysis, tonsillectomy etc.

Causes. Acute gastritis, gastric ulcer, carcinoma, oesophageal varices, splenic anaemia, leukaemia, overdosage of anticoagulants, septicaemia, trauma.

Signs and symptoms. Sudden onset of vomiting dark red or brown fluid (blood altered by gastric juice); rapid pulse; falling blood pressure; pallor; sweating; weakness; fainting; nausea; anxiety.

Treatment. As for haemorrhage in duodenal ulcer.

Perforation. Erosion through stomach wall with spilling of contents into peritoneal cavity.

Signs and symptoms. As for perforation in duodenal ulcer. Definite association with emotional or physical stress. Ten times more common in men than women.

Treatment. Immediate surgical closure.

Hour-glass stomach. Scar tissue contracts as gastric ulcer heals dividing stomach into two cavities. Rare, Symptoms similar to pyloric stenosis.

Pyloric stenosis. Ulcer heals near pyloric antrum and scar tissue contracts. Similar condition to pyloric obstruction in carcinoma of stomach.

Signs and symptoms. Pain due to violent peristalsis; vomiting; rapid loss of weight; splashing sounds on movement and on palpation of epigastrium; palpable mass at pylorus. Later copious vomiting and contains food eaten previous day.

Later — dehydration — dry skin, sunken eyes. Blood urea rises. May be tetany due to chloride loss in vomit.

Diagnosis. Fasting juice greater than 50 ml. Barium meal shows dilated stomach and overactive peristalsis.

Treatment. Partial gastrectomy with gastro-jejunostomy.

Infantile (congenital) pyloric stenosis

Hypertrophy and spasm of pyloric sphincter.

Cause. Unknown. More common in baby boys than girls (5:1).

Signs and symptoms. Sudden onset of projectile vomiting in a previously healthy babe; occurs about 10th day. Rapid dehydration, wasting; tetanic convulsions due to chloride loss; palpable tumour to right of umbilicus; visible peristalsis; constipation.

Treatment. Correct dehydration and electrolyte imbalance by intravenous infusion. Fredet-Ramstedt operation performed — hypertrophied circular fibres of pyloric sphincter cut through but mucous membrane left intact.

In some cases vomiting may not occur after every feeding. This may be due to pylorospasm rather than hypertrophy of sphincter. In such cases operation may be unnecessary. An antispasmodic drug such as methyl atropine nitrate (Eumydrine) 5 ml, 1 in 10 000 solution, orally half an hour before, then slow and careful feeding with thickened feeds may be sufficient.

Cancer of stomach

Signs and symptoms. Most common form of cancer of digestive tract. Occurs most commonly in males over 40 years. Incidence declining over last 15 years. Early symptoms are slight and patient unwilling to seek medical advice with trivial complaints. Often symptoms resemble those of peptic ulcer and treatment for same may be effective at first. Later — loss of weight; pain increasing in intensity and not related to taking food; haematemesis, melaena; occult blood in stools; anaemia.

Diagnosis. Gastric acid diminished or absent in 75 per cent of cases even after histamin challenge. Barium may show irregularity of gastric filling, altered motility, unusual mucosal pattern. Gastroscopy with biopsy of suspicious mass.

Treatment. Exploratory laparotomy and excision of mass if metastases have not occurred. Occasionally, when inoperable, a palliative short circuit operation may prevent death by starvation.

Dumping syndrome

Sudden onset of symptoms suggestive of shock about ½–1 hour after a meal. Occurs only in patients who have had gastric operations — partial gastrectomy, short circuits, etc.

Cause. Not known. May be rapid release of insulin when meal contains large amounts of carbohydrate.

Signs and symptoms. Pallor; weakness; fainting; rapid pulse; low blood pressure; sweating.

Treatment. During attack. Rest flat with foot of bed raised or feet raised. *Prevention.* Small frequent meals as in peptic ulcer; keep carbohydrate contents of each meal as low as possible; eat slowly, chewing well and swallowing small amounts at a time.

The intestines: diseases of the intestines

Bacillary dysentery

A specific infectious disease characterised by vomiting, diarrhoea and colicky pain.

Cause. Shigella organisms. (*S. sonne; S. flexner; S. shiga.*)

Pathology. General inflammation of mucous membrane of stomach and intestines which may become localized in ileum, caecum and ascending colon. Ulceration of mucous membranes leads to pus, mucus and blood in stools.

Spread. Carriers and flies contaminate water and milk supplies.

Signs and symptoms. May be mild and pass unreported. Abrupt onset of diarrhoea, tenesmus, nausea and vomiting. Malaise; aching of joints and muscles; abdominal cramp and waves of colic; pyrexia may be severe: 40°C. In children — rapid dehydration and prostration.

Treatment. Isolate patient; correct dehydration and electrolyte imbalance with intravenous fluids — saline, glucose, Hartmann's solution; maintain urinary output at 1½ litres minimum per day. *Specific drugs.* Sulphadiazine, sulphasuxidine; for strains resistant to sulphas broad spectrum antibiotics — tetracyclines, chloramphenicol, ampicillin. Specific antitoxins available.

Great care needed to ensure efficient current disinfection of all items from sick room. *Diet.* After initial correction of dehydration patient should be encouraged to take large amounts of fluid

— clear soups, albumin water, barley water, weak tea, fruit juices (fresh and strained), jellies. Proceed to mashed potatoes, milky dishes, lightly boiled or poached eggs, steamed fish, chicken, strained vegetables. Patient should not return to full normal diet for 6–8 weeks.

Nursing care includes careful oral hygiene, prevention of pressure sores, application of soothing creams to anus. *Complications*. Perforation. Haemorrhage. Acute arthritis. Excoriation of anus. Renal failure due to dehydration.

Infantile gastro-enteritis

A form of dysentery occurring in children under 2 years.

Cause. Certain strains of *Escherichia coli* (colon bacillus). Also secondary to many infectious diseases — pneumonia, measles, diphtheria. No definite organisms isolated from stools in many instances. Growing evidence for viral infection in many outbreaks.

Signs and symptoms. Abrupt onset with vomiting, colicky pain, diarrhoea, swelling of abdomen with gas (tympanites). Rapid dehydration with sunken eyes, sagging cheeks, inelastic skin, depressed fontanelles. General toxaemia with ashen grey complexion, restlessness; later — torpor and, possibly, coma and death.

Treatment. Strict isolation nursing. Correct dehydration and electrolyte imbalance promptly by intravenous fluids. (Frequently veins are small and collapsed in these babes and subcutaneous infusion performed instead). Antibiotics contraindicated if specific organisms not isolated.

Diet. Milk feeds should be stopped and boiled water substituted. When diarrhoea lessens oral fluids should be tried — isotonic saline/dextrose mixture. If no diarrhoea babe may progress through ¼ strength milk, to ½ strength, to ¾ strength and back to full strength on successive days.

Food poisoning

Diarrhoea and/or vomiting from eating food contaminated with chemical poison, preformed bacterial toxin or live bacteria, or poisonous natural vegetation, e.g. berries, fungi.

Cause. Poor hygiene in preparation, handling, storage or distribution of food especially cooked meats, 'ready-to-eat' dishes — custards, milky dishes etc. Organisms which produce toxins under such conditions are staphylococci, streptococci and salmonella. *Clostridium botulinum* needs special conditions — insufficient sterilisation of food or containers, an alkaline or neutral medium and sealing down to exclude oxygen — as in bottling or canning.

Signs and symptoms. Onset of colicky pain, nausea, vomiting and diarrhoea 1–50 hours after ingesting contaminated food. Often occurs in epidemic form among persons who have all eaten one particular item of food — many cases occurring within hours of each other. General symptoms vary in intensity — malaise, aching joints and muscles.

Treatment. Withhold food. Stomach lavage of doubtful value unless cause is traced to a meal taken not more than 3 hours before. Analgesics to reduce pain if severe. Maintain fluid balance intravenously if vomiting persists and prevents oral intake. Most cases recover in 1–3 days. In *Clostridium botulinum* infection (botulism) condition may be rapidly fatal. The toxin is extraordinarily powerful and affects the nerves causing paralysis, respiratory and cardiac failure. Botulinus antitoxin effective in early stages.

Crohn's disease (*regional ileitis*)

Inflammatory condition of gastro-intestinal tract affecting any part of digestive tract — more common in terminal ileum.

Cause. Unknown. Affects both sexes and all ages but most common between 20–40 years. Women more than men. Some evidence for viral cause.

Pathology. Usually chronic but may appear in acute form. Inflammatory process involves whole thickness of intestinal wall. Usually begins beneath mucosa and spreads through muscle coat to peritoneum. Ulcerates mucosa. Initial lesion in 15–30 cm of terminal ileum. May spread back up small intestine or on into caecum and colon. May 'skip' a distance and begin another lesion some segments away. Affected parts become thickened and lumen narrowed.

Signs and symptoms. Very variable depending on site affected. Pain in right iliac fossa similar to appendicitis; diarrhoea; history of intestinal colic; abdominal mass may be felt; weight loss; pyrexia; anaemia; occult blood in stools. Anal fistula occurs in high percentage of cases.

Diagnosis. Barium meal with follow-through and enema — shows narrowed segments or, in advanced cases, strictures and fistulae. Sigmoidoscopy. Colonoscopy. Biopsy.

Need to distinguish from tuberculosis, lymphoma, carcinoma, ulcerative colitis.

Complications. Intestinal obstruction. Fistula formation. Abscesses. Perforation. Steatorrhoea. Ankylosing spondylitis (cause unknown).

Treatment. No cure. May 'burn' itself out. Recurrence with or without treatment is common. *Medical*: Diet — maintain nutrition, high calorie, low residue, bland, vitamin and iron supplements. Rest — prolonged — fever tends to settle. Drugs — corticosteroids — usually reserved for seriously ill patients preoperatively. Antibiotics — of doubtful value.

Sulphasalazine (Salazopyrin) useful for acute disease. Some patients respond to azathioprine (Imuran). Metronidazole (Flagyl) often improves condition if fistulae and perianal complications present.

Surgical. Indications — strictures causing obstructions, failure to respond to medical therapy, management of complications.

Resection of strictures with end-to-end anastomosis. Split ileostomy allows local instillation of corticosteroids into colon and continuity may be restored at future date.

Prognosis. Most patients maintained in reasonably good health but recurrence and complications occur in 50 per cent within ten years.

Coeliac disease

Allergic disease characterized by intestinal sensitivity to gluten which occurs in wheat. Malabsorption of many other food factors follows — vitamin B_{12}, iron, fats, the fat soluble vitamins A, D, K, calcium, protein, carbohydrates — hence symptoms may be of several conditions — anaemia, dwarfism, tetany, rickets etc.

Signs and symptoms. Onset in childhood and persisting into adult life if untreated. Passage of bulky fatty stools coinciding with weaning and introduction of farinaceous foods. Wretchedly unhappy child with anorexia, failure to thrive, absence of subcutaneous fat with swollen abdomen and loose dry skin. Blood tests show reduction in calcium and phosphates; softening of bones and coeliac rickets result. X-ray with barium shows dilated small intestine. Duodenal biopsy shows flattened villi, absent microvilli, monocytic infiltration of mucosa. Repeat after treatment shows resumption of normal pattern.

Treatment. Dietary. Exclude all products containing wheat flour — bread, biscuits, cakes, semolina, pasta (spaghetti, macaroni, vermicelli etc.) tinned foods, sausages, ice-cream, malted milk and Ovaltine, sauces, gravies. Normal protein and fat is given and bread substitutes made with wheat starch. Milk and cornflour, beans and fresh vegetables provide sufficient variety. Rice. Maize. Soya flour.

Careful record of weight should show normal progress.

Complications. Lymphoma of jejunum. Ulceration. Malabsorption may continue in spite of gluten free diet.

Appendicitis

Inflammation of appendix occurring most commonly in children and young adults. Narrow lumen of appendix may become occluded due to oedema of its mucous lining. Anything trapped distal to blockage may undergo bacterial decomposition. Toxic absorption causes general symptoms. Contiguous spread may cause peritonitis.

Signs and symptoms. Pain starts in umbilical region, later moves to right iliac fossa; mild and intermittent at first, becoming severe and continuous later. Anorexia, nausea and vomiting — generally mild. Constipation common — occasionally diarrhoea. Tenderness marked in right iliac fossa — position of maximum tenderness over McBurney's point, one third of distance from anterior superior iliac spine to umbilicus. As irritation of peritoneum spreads, tenderness becomes more generalized with rigidity (guarding) of abdominal muscles. Tenderness on rectal and vaginal examination. General symptoms — low fever, leucocytosis.

Treatment. Close observation until diagnosis certain then prompt surgical removal. Rest in bed; nil orally; no laxatives or enemata which stimulate peristalsis and may cause perforation; no sedatives or analgesics which would mask signs and symptoms. If surgery not possible, antibiotics may be used. Ochsner-Sherren regime — nurse sitting up to encourage drainage of pus to pelvis; observations taken and charted ½–1 hourly;

most important sign — increasing pulse rate. Fluid balance chart. Observe stools for mucus (pelvic abscess). Intravenous fluids if patient unable to take oral fluids. No food. Morphia for pain. No laxatives or enemata for 3 days then suppositories. Under this treatment peritonitis should resolve but rising pulse rate and increase in pain may indicate that surgery is imperative.

Complications. Perforation with generalized peritonitis. Gangrene and severe toxic absorption. Appendix abscess. Portal pyaemia. Thrombosis of mesenteric veins. Sub-phrenic abscess. Adhesions and subsequent intestinal obstruction.

Appendix abscess

Pathology. Omentum and loops of small bowel become matted together round inflamed appendix and partition the area from general peritoneal cavity. Abscess forms in centre of mass.

Signs and symptoms. 2–6 days after onset — malaise, pallor, swinging pyrexia, leucocytosis, tender mass palpable in right iliac fossa.

Treatment. Ochsner-Sherren treatment as above. Outline mass in right iliac fossa each day — should become smaller. If abscess resolves, perform appendicectomy 6–12 weeks later. If signs persist and mass gets bigger — incise and drain.

Paralytic ileus

Stasis of small bowel varying in extent and duration.

Cause. Disturbance of Auerbach's and Meissner's plexuses due to trauma, surgical handling of gut, peritonitis, pancreatitis, mesenteric thrombosis and embolism. Spinal injuries (disturbance of sympathetic system).

Signs and symptoms. Discomfort; distension, vomiting — first stomach contents, then bile stained fluid, lastly large quantities of brownish foul smelling fluid — faecal vomit — leading to dehydration, electrolyte imbalance. Absence of bowel sounds. Abdomen distended but soft. X-ray shows loops of intestines dilated with gas.

Treatment. Nothing by mouth. Correct dehydration and electrolyte imbalance with intravenous fluids. Keep stomach empty by aspirating hourly through Ryle's tube. Miller-Abbott tube may be employed — long rubber tube with double lumen and inflatable balloon near tip. Tube passed into stomach, balloon inflated, withdrawn against cardiac sphincter, balloon deflated.

With patient lying on right side tube passed a further 35 cm. It will pass into duodenum and can be passed into small intestine. Re-inflation of balloon helps this. Peristalsis carries it to paralysed section. Attachment to a low pressure pump keeps intestines deflated and empty and assists recovery.

Recovery heralded by absence of aspirate, resumption of bowel sounds and passage of flatus. Cautious reintroduction of diet may then start.

Mesenteric lymphadenitis

Recurrent attacks of inflammation of one or more groups of mesenteric glands.

Signs and symptoms. Recurrent abdominal pain, mild pyrexia, occasionally diarrhoea, nausea, vomiting. Pain often maximal in right iliac fossa but not sharply localized at McBurney's point. Pain constant and not collicky. PR tenderness not excessive. Often recent history of upper respiratory infections.

Often diagnosed as appendicitis but appendix normal at operation and condition recurs later.

Treatment. Observation to differentiate from appendicitis, renal tract infection, nil specific.

Meckel's diverticulum

Persistence of duct which in fetus connects yolk sac to intestine.

Pathology. Occurs in 2 per cent of population. Pouch about 5 cm long opens into ileum about 1 m above ileocaecal junction. Lumen same width as ileum. Blind end may be free or attached to abdominal wall or intestines by fibrous cord. Mucous lining may contain functional gastric or pancreatic cells.

Signs and symptoms. Usually asymptomatic. May develop painless peptic ulcer which is revealed by haemorrhage or perforation. May cause obstruction by adhesions or intussusception. If inflamed, may resemble appendicitis.

Treatment. Surgical — laparotomy and excision.

Large intestine: diseases of the colon and rectum

Ulcerative colitis

Chronic ulcerative condition of large intestine.

Cause. Unknown. Possible viral.

Signs and symptoms. Diarrhoea. Frequent stools contain

blood, mucus and pus. Fever; dehydration; prostration; rapid loss of weight; anaemia. Spontaneous recovery occurs but relapses are common.

Diagnosis. Sigmoidoscopy. Barium enema. Stool culture reveals no pathogens. Mucous membrane oedematous, reddened, blood vessel pattern obliterated. Contact bleeding occurs when membrane lightly swabbed. In long standing cases granulations occur producing warty outgrowths called pseudopolypi. Barium enema shows loss of haustrations and a narrowed, shortened colon.

Treatment. Medical. During severe acute attacks patient admitted. Corticosteroids administered at once, intravenously in very severe cases, otherwise orally and locally, e.g. cortisone 200 mg b.d.; ACTH 80 U b.d.; prednisolone 20 mg daily. Suppositories or enema avoids systemic reactions.

Diet — high calorie high protein, high fibre with iron and vitamin supplements. A few cases respond to milk free diet.

Dehydration and electrolyte imbalance corrected by i.v. fluids.

Less severe cases treated at home with prednisolone 20 mg daily, daily enema of prednisolone 20 mg in 100 ml (Predsol) for 4–6 weeks.

Remissions maintained with Sulphasalazine (Salazopyrine) 2 g orally daily, indefinitely.

Others used azothioprine (Imuran) for patients failing to respond to sulphasalazine. Sodium chomoglycate (Nalcrom) experimental.

Surgery. Indications include failure to respond to medical treatment, development of complications, perforation, carcinoma, stricture.

Proctocolectomy with ileostomy gives best results.

Complications. Perforation. Haemorrhage. Malignant change. Large bowel obstruction following healing. Ischio-rectal abscess. Fistulae. Arthritis. Iritis. Mouth ulceration.

Diverticulosis

Associated with low faecal volume due to lack of fibre and other indigestible residue in food. Intra-colonic pressure needed to propel small hard faecal masses. Muscular layers hypertrophy, causing narrowing of lumen and intermittent obstruction.

Diverticulae balloon out from wall. Unlikely that inflammatory reaction occurs in diverticulae to cause 'diverticulitis' unless perforation and peri-colic abscess occurs.

Signs and symptoms. Occurs mainly in individuals over 40 years. Abdominal pain and tenderness over site — right side must be differentiated from appendicitis. Constipation common.

Diagnosis. Sigmoidoscopy may visualize diverticula. Narrowing and fixation of the recto-sigmoid junction common. Barium enema often shows position and number of diverticula.

Treatment. High residue diet and anti-constipation measures. Antibiotics during acute attack — penicillin 600 000 units and streptomycin 0·5 g twice daily. Bulk residue increased with Normocol, Fibogel.

Severe diverticulitis needs admission, stomach aspiration, i.v. fluid replacement, pethidine, antibiotics, observation to detect complications needing surgery.

Complications. Localized abscess formation. Perforation. Adherence to nearby organs especially bladder. Fistulae. Acute intestinal obstruction from adherent bands. Chronic intestinal obstruction from thickening of wall with fibrous tissue.

Irritable bowel syndrome

Periodic attacks of left iliac fossa colic with alteration of bowel habit. More common in females of 20–30 years.

Symptoms similar to diverticulosis but investigations — digital examination, sigmoidoscopy, barium enema — show nothing abnormal. Important to exclude carcinoma.

Treatment similar to that for diverticular disease — high residue diet supplemented with bulk producing agents as Normacol or Fibogel.

Hirschsprung's disease

Congenital absence of Meissner's and Auerbach's plexuses in wall of part or all of colon leading to inefficient peristalsis and gross dilatation and hypertrophy of colon.

Signs and symptoms. Constipation from childhood. Gross abdominal distension. Child pale and toxaemic.

Diagnosis. Barium enema — very large quantity of barium needed to fill colon. Descending and sigmoid colon especially dilated. Biopsy of rectal wall shows derangement of nerve net and absence of ganglion cells.

Treatment. Diagnosis should be attempted at youngest age possible. Biopsy performed in any baby who has severe constipation. Laparotomy performed before onset of compensatory hypertrophy and dilatation of normal gut proximal to deranged area. Rectosigmoid resection and anastomosis at anus (pull-through operation) gives good chance of normal life. In established cases keep colon empty with daily enema, abdominal massage, daily liquid paraffin to keep stools soft. Aperients not used. Spinal anaesthesia relaxes anal sphincter and permits initial emptying of colon.

Colostomy or ileostomy may be necessary if diagnosis made after dilatation occurs.

Carcinoma of colon and rectum

Signs and symptoms. Change in bowel habits. Alternating constipation and diarrhoea. Mucoid or bloody stools. Cramping abdominal pain. Anaemia. Weight loss. Carcinoma of left colon more likely to cause total obstruction which may be acute.

Diagnosis. Palpation per rectum. Sigmoidoscopy and biopsy. Barium enema. Laporotomy.

Treatment. Excision, preferably with anastomosis. Colostomy.

Haemorrhoids

Definition. Laxness of anal mucous membrane which allows haemorrhoidal veins to protrude into lumen of anus. Three main groups of vessels, left lateral, right posterior, right anterior (3 o'clock, 7 o'clock, 11 o'clock) form most of varices. Minor groups also present which may form varices.

Contributing factors. Constipation. Straining at stool. Pregnancy. Raised portal pressure. Hereditary factor.

Signs and symptoms. Intermittent anal discomfort rarely amounting to pain unless prolapsed. Pruritis ani. Prolapse. Bleeding which may be persistent and sometimes severe.

Diagnosis. Inspection. Proctoscopy. Other causes of rectal bleeding must be excluded, e.g. polyps, carcinoma, fissure.

Complications. Anaemia. Infection. Prolapse. Strangulation. Ulceration. Thrombosis.

Treatment. (1) Conservative. Avoidance of constipation with high residue diet, stool softeners such as mineral oil. Early reduction of prolapse. Application of anaesthetic cream or suppository half hour before bowel action. (2) Surgical. Ligation and careful dissection of haemorrhoids individually. Injection of sclerosing agent around base of early pile may help to prevent slippage of mucous membrane thought by many to be prime cause of condition.

Liver

Liver function tests

Serum bilirubin (Van den Bergh reaction). Normally only fat soluble bilirubin (haemobilirubin) present in blood. In some types of jaundice, water soluble bilirubin (hepatobilirubin) passes back into the blood and can be detected. Bilirubin in blood can be expressed in 3 ways:

1. By weight — normal amount present 6–24 micromoles/l.
2. By dilution strength — normal 1 part in 1 000 000 to 1 in 400 000.
3. In units taking 1 part in 200 000 as 1 unit —normal 0·2–0·5 units.

Bromsulphthalein test (BSP). Measures excretory power of liver. BSP 5 mg/kg in 5 per cent saline injected intravenously. 1 hour later amount in blood measured. Normally all excreted.

Flocculation tests. Abnormal forms of albumin and globulin made by diseased liver cells. Serum set up against various salts — gold, thymol, cephalin, cholesterol — presence of abnormal proteins results in cloudiness (flocculation).

Galactose test. 40 g galactose in 50 ml water taken after fasting. 5 hours later urine collected. If it contains 2 g or more galactose liver damage indicated.

Vitamin K response. Low prothrombin in blood may be due to: (1) lack of absorption of vitamin K (obstructive jaundice); (2) failure to utilize vitamin K (toxic jaundice). After injection of vitamin K serum prothrombin rises in obstructive jaundice, in toxic jaundice level remains depressed.

Serum albumen. Almost all produced by liver. Normal value 3·3 to 6:5 g/100 ml.

Serum enzymes. SGOT Normal 5 — 40 iu/100 ml SGPT 5 — 35 iu/100 ml. LDH. Gamma GT.

Jaundice
Retention of bilirubin within the body.

Types. 1. Haemolytic. Bilirubin released into blood faster than liver can convert it to water soluble form.

2. Toxic. Liver cells, damaged by disease or toxins, allow return of altered bilirubin to blood stream.

3. Obstructive. Water soluble form of bilirubin cannot escape into intestine.

Haemolytic jaundice. Caused by excessive blood destruction. (See haemolytic anaemia p. 33). *Toxic jaundice*. Hepatitis. Damages liver cells. (1) viral: (2) chemical poisons — trinitrotoluene, tetrachlorethane, chlorine gas, arsenic, phosphorus, chloroform; (3) toxins of any micro-organisms in severe infections; (4) malaria; (5) toxaemia of pregnancy. *Obstructive jaundice*. Obstruction of bile ducts — gallstones, parasitic worms (rarely). Thickening of wall of duct — carcinoma, postoperative stenosis, trauma. Pressure outside duct — carcinoma head of pancreas. Congenital atresia of bile ducts.

Signs and symptoms. Due to increased bilirubin in blood stream and decreased bilirubin in intestines.

Colour of skin and mucous membranes varies from pale lemon to deep orange-bronze. Detected earliest in conjunctiva. Urine — darkens, froths readily forming yellow bubbles, contains bile stained casts and albumin (urine normal in haemolytic jaundice as unaltered bilirubin does not pass into nephrons). Faeces — bulky, greasy, clay coloured, foul smelling. (Normal in haemolytic jaundice as liver is excreting bilirubin as fast as it can). Itching may be severe and difficult to allay. Low prothrombin level in blood due to lack of absorption from intestine of vitamin K in absence of bile. Mental depression and irritability. Yellow vision when heavily jaundiced. Anorexia. Nausea. Intolerance of fatty foods.

Treatment. Basically — treat the underlying cause. Itching may be relieved by cool sodium bicarbonate baths — 100 g sodium bicarbonate added to bath water at 37°C.; calamine lotion. Stools, urine and skin return to normal as jaundice abates. Fats are poorly tolerated and should be omitted from diet in obstructive jaundice due to blockage of common bile duct by gall stone — fats stimulate production of cholecystokinin which causes contractions of gallbladder. Vitamin K given when prothrombin level reduce, 5–25 mg intramuscularly or intravenously, dose depending on reduction.

Diseases of the liver

Viral (infective) hepatitis

Infectious disease causing cellular damage to liver.

Cause. Virus A or IH which is isolated from patient's faeces and serum by growth on tissue culture and chick embryo.

Transmission. Faecal contamination of food and water by patient, carriers, flies.

Incubation period. 2–6 weeks.

Course. Most cases recover completely and are immune from further attacks. Irritability and mental depression may persist for many weeks. Occasionally severe liver damage and failure. Occasionally cirrhosis of liver.

Signs and symptoms. Fever 38·3–39·4°C with headache, weakness, joint pains, resembling influenza. Anorexia, nausea, vomiting, diarrhoea. Urine darkens first, then faeces become pale, then skin darkens. Jaundice — variable, may be absent or may be the only sign. Pain — variable, often absent, may be severe in right side and back.

Diagnosis. Confirmed by liver function tests. Serum bilirubin raised; serum prothrombin depressed; serum transaminase raised; flocculation tests positive. Where facilities available, virus may be isolated from serum or faeces.

Treatment. Rest in bed while febrile. Thereafter, activity reduced but confinement to bed contra-indicated. Diet rich in glucose and first class proteins. Fats not specially contra-indicated but patient often dislikes them. Avoid drugs metabolized by liver (barbiturates, morphia, sulphonamides, alcohol) to prevent further cellular damage. Long convalescence in restful environment advised.

Serum hepatitis (Homologous serum jaundice)

Caused by virus B or SH. Spread only by contact or inoculation with human blood products. Incubation period 6 weeks — 6 months. Infection can be severe, even fatal. It is estimated that 2–3 per cent of world adult population are carriers of virus B or SH.

Signs, symptoms and treatment are the same as for infective hepatitis. Often history of infections. Common in drug addicts.

Serological fluorescent tests show presence of Australia antigen in Heptatitis B. Great care needed in handling any secretions from such patients, especially blood, syringes and needles.

Drug hepatitis

Liver cell damage due to drugs which are metabolized by liver.

Causes. Chloramphenicol. Tetracyclines. Phenylbutazone. Phenothiazides. Chlorpropamide. Chlorothiazide. Erythromycin.

Signs and symptoms. Very similar to viral hepatitis.

Treatment. Withdraw drug at once. Give diet rich in glucose and first class proteins.

(Cortisone is not generally given in any form of hepatitis unless symptoms worsen and patient in danger of acute liver failure).

Leptospirosis (Weil's disease. Spirochaetal jaundice)

General febrile illness, more prevalent than previously thought. (Most cases mild and undiagnosed).

Cause. Spirochaetes — from rats (*Leptospira icterohaemorrhagiae*); from dogs (*L. canicola*); from cows and pigs (*L. pomona*).

Spread. Urine of infected animals contaminate food, drinking water, washing water, swimming pools, sewers, canals. Organism can penetrate unbroken skin.

Signs and symptoms. Very variable. Mild cases — low pyrexia, slight jaundice. Severe cases — hepatitis, nephritis, purpura, meningitis.

Diagnosis. Examination of blood and urine for organisms — animal inoculation with centrifuge deposit for urine. Agglutination test positive after 7th day of illness.

Treatment. Tetracycline 0.5 g 6 hourly for 6 days, or procaine penicillin 1 megaunit intramuscularly daily $\times$ 7 days.

Renal failure requires dialysis. Good prognosis.

Cirrhosis of the liver

Chronic and slowly progressive destruction of liver cells. Normal liver lobules surrounded and isolated by fibrous tissue. Nodular regeneration of hepatocytes without the orderly arrangement of portal tracts, biliary canaliculi and hepatic vessel.

Portal obstruction and liver failure occurs.

Cause. Unknown.

Contributory factors. Chronic protein deficiency. Vitamin B complex deficiency. Alcoholism. Repeated poisoning with hepatotoxic drugs. Congenital syphilis. Repeated attacks of malaria. Acute hepatitis.

Age of onset. 40 years and upwards. Males more commonly than females (2:1).

Signs and symptoms. Jaundice. Pruritus. Insidious onset with muscle weakness, exercise intolerance, anorexia, weight loss, nausea, vomiting, alternating bouts of diarrhoea and constipation, loss of sexual desire, impotence, sterility. Skin becomes red with groups of dilated visible capillaries. Palms mottled. Hepatic and splenic enlargement. Oesophageal and gastric varices. Haemorrhoids.

Later — fever; lower limb oedema and ascites; hydrothorax; haematemesis; dilated veins of neck and abdomen.

Very late — tremor, sluggish pupils, delirium, drowsiness. Arteriosclerosis and myocarditis common.

Diagnosis. Bromsulphtalein test positive. Liver biopsy shows deteriorated cells. Oesophagosopy or barium meals shows oesophageal varices. Liver function tests show raised SGOT, LDH, alkaline phosphatase, bilirubin. Serum albumen decreased.

Treatment. No cure but strictly ordered life keeps patient in reasonable health for many years. 10 hours in bed at night. Rest periods during day. No alcohol. No smoking. High protein diet — 1·5 g/kg per day, all first class protein. Vitamin B complex supplements.

Ascites and oedema may be due to sodium retention — reduce sodium intake to 1 g daily (no added salt). Give diuretics — chlorothiazide and spironolactone. Paracentesis only if painful and uncomfortable.

Many later symptoms caused by inability of liver to deal with ammonia. Much of this produced in and absorbed from bowel. Greater risk of this on high protein diet or if there is blood in the bowel. Control by temporarily reducing protein intake and clearing bowel of blood as rapidly as possible after haematemesis etc. — milk of magnesia 30 ml 4 times daily. Fungal activity in bowel also produces ammonia — reduce fungi with neomycin

0·75 g 6 hourly for 6 days. Argenine therapy — argenine is a hexose base amino acid which replaces ammonia in the blood. 500 ml 5 per cent argenine hydrochloride in 10 per cent glucose intravenously given in 2 hours, repeat 8–12 hourly (may be ineffective in chronic hepatic insufficiency).

Anaemia — ferrous sulphate (enteric coated) 200–300 mg thrice daily.

Haematemesis may be severe. Sengstaken triple lumen tube may be effective. Balloon applies pressure to wall of oesophagus and allows gastric suction for removal of blood, washout and feeding. Blood transfusion as indicated. Vitamin K 5–25 mg by injection depending on depression of serum prothrombin (may be ineffective in severe cirrhosis).

Surgery may be performed in severe portal hypertension. Anastomosis of portal vein to inferior vena cava. Poor risk.

Portal hypertension
  Definition. Persistent portal pressure over 20 mmHg.
  Cause. Obstruction of portal venous system.
  (1) Pre-sinusoidal — thrombosis, new growths, cirrhotic fibrosis, schistosomiasis.
  (2) Post-sinusoidal.
    Budd-Chiari syndrome.
    Vena caval webbing.
  Results. Development of collateral circulation with systemic circulation increasing pressure within submucous oesophageal veins, oesophageal varices.
  Splenic congestion leading to thrombocytopenia, leucopenia and anaemia. Ascites. Hepatic coma. Encephalopathy.
  Signs and symptoms. May be overshadowed by symptoms of primary condition. Often not diagnosed until oesophageal varices displayed on X-ray, or haemorrhage occurs.
  Other systemic veins subject to dilation — haemorrhoids, periumbilical, abdominal wall, retroperitoneal space. All may bleed. Splenomegaly.
  Diagnosis. Barium swallow. Oesophagoscopy. Portal venography.
  Treatment. Prompt resuscitation following bleeding — transfusion with fresh blood, possibly fresh frozen plasma and platelet — rich concentrate.

Bowel should be cleared of blood to reduce chance of hepatic coma — enema, gastric suction.

Sterilize bowel with oral Neomycin.

Vasopressin causes splanchnic vasoconstriction. Given iv. 20 U hourly, in 5 per cent glucose.

Balloon tamponade by Sengstaken tube effective in short term.

Surgical measures may be needed if bleeding persists — ligation of varices directly or reduction of portal pressure by various shunt techniques.

Hydatid cyst

Infestation with ova of dog tapeworm (*Taenia echninococcus*) which forms a cyst in liver (occasionally other organs).

Life cycle of parasite. Active tapeworm stage in intestines of dogs, wolves, coyotes, etc. Worm is 3–6 mm mm long with only 3 segments. May exist in vast numbers in intestine. Ova passed in faeces and may contaminate pastureland, water etc. Intermediate hosts — practically any warm blooded animal especially sheep. Ova ingested and carried to liver by portal circulation. May pass into general circulation. Man usually infected by household pets.

Pathology. Usually single cyst develops. Cyst wall double layered, inner layer grows heads (scolices) of new tapeworms, outer layer chitinous and tends to become calcified in man. Parts of inner layer may become dislodged and form daugher cysts within parent cyst. If cyst wall breaks, satellite cysts may form in liver. If cyst ruptures into peritoneal cavity severe anaphylactic shock results from liberation of toxic material.

Signs and symptoms. Symptoms vary according to site of cyst. In liver simulates malignant growth; in brain — cerebral tumour; in lungs — compression and pleural fluid.

In liver, causes symptomless swelling. Later — pain in right side often referred to shoulder. Biliary colic and jaundice may occur if cyst ruptures into biliary passages. Allergic reactions if cyst bursts — urticaria, gastro-intestinal disturbance, eosinophilia, anaphylactic shock. Rarely peritonitis.

Diagnosis. Confirmed by eosinophilia and positive Casoni tent (0·5 to 1 ml sterilized hydatid fluid injected intradermally. Positive reaction — area of erythema with central weal develops within 10 minutes). Results 75–95 per cent accurate. Complement fixation test more intricate but 100 per cent accurate.

Course of disease. (1) Parasite dies, fluid absorbed and cyst calcified (2) Surgical removal when diagnosed. (3) Cyst ruptures causing allergic reaction and growth of satellite cysts. (4) Rarely, infection of cyst causing liver abscess.

Treatment. Surgical removal. Attempt made to excise complete cyst without causing it to rupture. If it ruptures exhaustive search made for any escaped daugher cysts before closing abdomen.

The gallbladder and bile ducts: diseases of gallbladder and bile ducts

Acute cholecystitis

Inflammation of gallbladder. 90 per cent of cases associated with gallstones, usually superimposed on chronic state.

Signs and symptoms. Sudden onset of severe pain in right hypochondrium radiating to right shoulder. Often occurs after a heavy meal. Rebound tenderness following sudden release of pressure over gallbladder area. Leucocytosis.

Diagnosis. Stones seen on X-ray in 25 per cent cases. Cholecystogram — gallbladder fails to fill.

Complications of untreated cases. Gangrene of gallbladder. Cholangitis. Perforation with peritonitis.

Treatment. During acute phase — rest in bed. Atropine 0·6 mg 4 hourly to reduce spasm. Meperidine (Demerol) 50–100 mg orally or by injection 3–4 hourly as an analgesics. (Morphia avoided as it induces spasm of sphincter of Oddi). Antibiotics — triple attack with penicillin, streptomycin and tetracycline.

Observe carefully for onset of complications which might need immediate surgery — increasing pain, rising temperature, increasing leucocytosis.

3 months after attack subsides — surgery. Cholecystectomy and exploration of bile ducts (Cholecystostomy in poor-risk patients).

Chronic cholecystitis

Causes. Infection usually with organisms of the enteric group, often *E. coli*. Also streptococci and staphylococci.

Signs and symptoms. Chronic dyspepsia, flatulence, nausea. Precipitated by fatty foods. Recurrent attacks of biliary colic — pain in right hypochondrium radiating to right shoulder lasting minutes or hours. Vomiting.

Diagnosis. Cholecystogram. X-ray may show stones.

Treatment. Surgery in good risk patients — cholecystectomy. Diet — non-greasy, no fried foods. Atropine 0·6 mg 4–6 hourly to relieve spasm. Sedation, phenobarbitone 30 mg 3 times daily.

Cholelithiasis

Stones in the gallbladder.

Causes. Function of gallbladder is to concentrate bile by absorbing nine tenths of its water. This alone is not sufficient to cause stones to form. Usually infectious factor involved. Cellular debris produced by bacteria acts as focus for deposition of solutes.

Types. Solutes — calcium salts, cholesterol, bile salts. Most stones mixture of all three. Usually multiple faceted stones.

Signs and symptoms. Most cases asymptomatic or vague until stone moves into cystic duct, then acute onset of biliary colic with chills and fever. Stone may move to duodenum, may move back into gallbladder, may block common bile duct causing jaundice and liver damage.

Complications. Liver damage, liver failure, portal obstruction, cholangitis, haemorrhage due to low prothrombin level.

Treatment. Dietary — high protein, high glucose, low fat, vitamin supplements, antibiotics. Serum prothrombin twice weekly and vitamin K injections to maintain prothrombin at normal level. Weekly liver function tests so that surgery can be performed before liver damage becomes serious.

Many surgeons advocate early surgery — cholecystectomy and exploration of bile ducts — because complications serious.

Cholangitis

Purulent inflammation of bile ducts.

Cause. Most commonly gallstones but can occur in any condition affecting the gallbladder.

Pathology. Dilated common bile duct with thickened walls. Liver enlarged and contains multiple small abscesses. Gallbladder — pus-filled bag (empyema). Adhesions and fistulae develop between gallbladder and nearby organs.

Signs and symptoms. Swinging temperature with rigors, nausea, vomiting. Severe jaundice. Pain and tenderness in right hypochondrium. Leucocytosis. Rapid weight loss.

Complications. Septicaemia. Pyaemia. Perforation. Peritonitis. Penetration and fistulae.

Treatment. Triple antibiotic therapy — penicillin, streptomycin, tetracycline.

Pancreas: disease of the pancreas

Pancreatic function tests

None highly specific.

1. Exocrine evaluation. Duodenal tube passed under X-ray control. Pancreatic secretion aspirated over timed period following i.v. injection of secretin or cholecystokinin or synthetic stimulant. Caerulein.

Alternatively secretion stimulated by test meal injected into stomach — 6 per cent fat, 15 per cent carbohydrate, 5 per cent protein in 300 ml water.

Aspirate tested for bicarbonate and enzyme content.

2. *Indirect tests*. Serum, faeces and urine may be examined for enzymes. Faecal chymotrypsin. Urinary trypsin. Serum polypepties.

Acute pancreatitis

Acute inflammation of pancreas with escape of enzymes into parenchyma and destruction of acinar cells.

Cause. Unknown. Some factor activates trypsinogen within pancreas. Commonly associated with alcoholism and gallstones.

Signs and symptoms. Sudden onset of severe abdominal pain radiating to back. Worse when lying flat. Relieved by sitting up. Nausea, vomiting, shock. Upper abdominal tenderness with muscle guarding. Leucocytosis. Albuminura. Glycosuria. Elevated blood sugar, serum amylase, urinary diastase.

Diagnosis. X-ray may show gallstones, upper portion of small intestine distended with gas, fluid in left pleural cavity.

Treatment. Immediate treatment for shock. Pethidine 100 mg 4 hourly. Intravenous therapy — 500 ml plasma then glucose saline as necessary. Continuous gastric suction. No oral foods or fluids temporarily. Vital signs observed and recorded every

15–30 minutes, temperature, pulse, blood pressure, haematocrit. Daily serum amylase, serum lipase, full blood count.

Often difficult to distinguish from perforated duodenal ulcer. After 48–72 hours oral fluids commenced. If tolerated, amount increased and diet started. Atropine continued 3 times daily to reduce pancreatic secretions.

Complications. Abscess. Pseudocyst. Diabetes.

Chronic relapsing pancreatitis

Series of less severe incidences. Often alcohol intake excessive. Eventually — pancreatic insufficiency and diabetes mellitus.

Carcinoma of pancreas

More common in males over 40 years. Head of pancreas most commonly affected.

Signs and symptoms. Constant pain in epigastrium. and left hypochondrium. Worse on lying flat, relieved when sitting up. Dyspepsia, anorexia, weight loss. Ampulla of Vater and common bile duct often involved early, causing jaundice. Liver enlarged. Metastases occur early. Diabetes mellitus especially if tail of pancreas involved.

Treatment. Most cases advanced when diagnosed. Surgical removal if possible. Palliative operation to provide a bypass for bile — cholecystojejunostomy.

Fibrocystic disease of the pancreas

One aspect of an hereditary disease in which mucous glands produce an extremely thick and viscid mucus. In the pancreas this blocks the ducts causing retention of pancreatic juice which forms cysts.

Cause. Unknown.

Signs and symptoms. In newborn — lack of pancreatic enzymes causes failure to mobilize meconium and intestinal obstruction results — meconium ileus. Treatment — operation to remove meconium. Second group — condition suspected after attack of staphylococcal pneumonia with atelectasis followed by poor digestion and rapid wasting. Resembles coeliac disease but appetite good.

Diagnosis. High output of chlorides in sweat. Petri dish prepared with agar, silver nitrate and potassium chromate. Child's palm pressed to this gives distinctive white print.

Intestinal juice shows absence of trypsin.

Treatment. Generous mixed diet with low fat content. Pancreatin (extract of pancreas containing enzymes) coated granules 1–2 g with meals. Guard against infections.

4. The Urinary System

Investigations of urinary system

X-ray

1. Simple X-ray. Plain radiograph may show outline of kidney but intestinal shadowing can obscure it. May show certain types of calculi, calcification due to tuberculosis or presence of abscess.

2. Intravenous urography (pyelography). Intravenous injection of radio-opaque substance that it excreted by kidneys. Films taken at appropriate intervals showing outlines of kidneys, pelves, ureters, bladder. (High blood urea prevents excretion of radio-opaque substance).

Preparation. Bowels must be clear of faeces and gas. Non-residue diet for 48 hours; fluids only during last 12 hours; aperient for 2 nights before; enema and rectal washout on morning of X-ray; patient encouraged to walk about and expel flatus.

3. Ureteric catheterization and retrograde pyelography. Cystoscope passed and uretic orifices visualized. Fine ureteric catheters passed, one into each ureter. Urine for examination can be collected separately from each kidney measuring rate of flow and amount passed. Opaque dye can be injected directly into kidney pelvis to give clear outline of calices.

Preparation. Same as for intravenous urography.

4. Nephrotomograph. Special X-rays taken after intravenous introduction of radio-opaque substance. These show kidney out of focus except at a set depth within its tissue. Series of such films with 'in focus' layer set at various depths allows a three dimensional impression to be built up. Shows extent of cysts, tubercular foci, cancer, calculi.

5. Arteriograph. Fine catheter passed via femoral artery into aorta and radio-opaque substance injected. As this flows through renal artery, X-rays taken to show any deformity of blood vessels.

6. Renal biopsy. Biopsy not carried out extensively until mid-century. Since then far greater understanding of lesions in glomerulonephritis and their relationship to ways in which disease presents has developed.

Clearance tests

Kidney ability can be measured by comparing the amount of certain substances in blood with that in urine passed during a known period. Result expressed as so much blood 'cleared' per minute, often turned into a percentage of the normal amount cleared.

Clearance of naturally occurring substances may be measured — urea, creatinine — or substances may be injected — inulin, para-aminohippuric acid.

Urea clearance is most common test. No restriction on diet and fluids before test. Patient drinks ½ litre of water half an hour before test begins to ensure reasonable urinary flow. Patient empties bladder completely, time noted. This specimen is not needed but time of passing is important. At exactly one hour intervals, patient empties bladder completely for three specimens. Exact time interval between specimens noted on labels and must be accurate to within one minute, otherwise false results occur. Blood sample taken about half way through test. Normal urea clearance is 75 ml blood cleared of urea per minute = 100 per cent. Lower figures indicate impairment of kidneys.

Concentration tests

These are designed to discover concentrating power of kidneys for certain substances. Most common substance used is urea. No fluids for 12 hours. Patient empties bladder completely at a certain hour, this specimen is discarded, but time is noted. He then drinks 15 g urea in 100 ml water. Urine passed at one hourly intervals for three specimens. Normally urea in the three specimens will rise above 2 g per 100 ml urine. If it remains constantly below 2 g per cent ability of kidney to concentrate urea is lowered.

Water concentration and dilution tests

When water is plentiful in body, tubules allow its escape in the urine. When the body is short of water the tubules allow less water to escape in urine. Amount of water in a specimen can be estimated by simply taking the specific gravity. A healthy person will pass urine of low specific gravity after drinking a lot and will pass urine of high specific gravity when intake reduced. Damaged kidneys lose this ability, urine passed is of fixed specific gravity irrespective of variation of intake.

Test may be a direct one in two parts. First patient drinks 2 litres of water in 20 minutes. Urine collected at hourly intervals for next 4 hours. Specific gravity taken each time, should fall to 1005 or lower. Total quantity measured. Almost all the 2 litres of water should be passed in 4 hours. In second part of test, fluids forbidden after 6 p.m. and urine collected at 8, 9 and 10 a.m. At least one of these specimens should have a specific gravity of 1020 or higher.

A simpler method of testing ability of kidney to concentrate is to inject 5 units of antidiuretic hormone. All urine passed in next 24 hours is saved and its specific gravity taken. At least once during the 24 hours reading should be over 1020.

Urine tests

Deposits. Microscopic examination of centrifuged deposits in urine may show red and white blood cells, crystals of various substances and casts (lining cells of tubules). In acute nephritis casts may be complete tubes. If casts have disintegrated, as in chronic kidney conditions, they are called granular or hyaline casts. *Urates.* Dirty white or pinkish deposit which disappears on boiling. *Phosphates.* White cloud, more obvious on boiling but disappears on adding acetic acid. *Uric acid.* Brick red deposit which disappears on boiling. *Pus.* Thick ropy sediment with an ammonia or fishy odour. *Mucus.* Thin flocculent deposit.

Reaction. Urine is usually acid but, not abnormally, can be alkaline especially after eating meals containing mainly vegetables. Acid turns litmus red, alkaline turns litmus blue. More delicate indicators used if exact degree of acidity required.

Specific gravity. Depends on amount of solutes. Normal range 1005 to 1025. Presistently high sp. gr. especially when large amounts of urine are passed indicates diabetes mellitus; persistently low sp. gr. indicates absence of urea; fixed sp. gr. at about 1010, in spite of variations of intake, indicates kidney damage.

Colour. Normal urine clear or very slightly cloudy and of yellow-brown colour. Other colours may indicate disease though not necessarily: black — phenol, melanin, haemoglobin; greenish brown — bile; dark red or brown — blood from high in the urinary tract; orange or red — carrots or beetroot eaten recently, blood from bladder or urethra, haemoglobin.

Dip stick urine tests have largely replaced lengthy chemical tests. Their ease of application, reliability and convenience have ensured universal use.

Collection of urine specimens

Early morning specimen. Patient asked to pass urine into clean receptacle on waking. This specimen more concentrated and more likely to contain abnormalities.

Mid-stream specimem. Vulva or penis thoroughly cleaned and dried. Patient given two containers and asked to direct urine stream first into one container, then into the other, and to finish off in first. Second container is sterile and contains required specimen. Care taken to avoid contamination.

Catheter specimen. Catheterization of patients merely to obtain specimen of urine avoided unless essential. Risk of infection high, especially in patients who have urinary conditions. When it must be performed utmost precautions taken.

Suprapubic puncture. With bladder full, lumbar puncture needle inserted over symphysis pubis and specimen aspirated. Less traumatic than catheterization and less risk of infection.

Twenty-four hour specimen. Patient empties bladder at certain hour and specimen discarded. All urine then saved until same time 24 hours later. Laboratory may need whole specimen or sample only. In latter case whole specimen shaken vigorously, whole amount measured and sample taken. Laboratory will want to know total amount.

Acute renal failure and dialysis: Acute renal failure

Sudden loss of ability to secrete urine.

Causes. 1. Blood pressure too low for kidneys to function — haemorrhage, shock, trauma, dehydration, burns. (Pre-renal causes). 2. Blockage of tubules — haemoglobin after mismatched blood transfusion, haemolysis in Weil's disease, malaria; myoglobin released from muscles following severe crush injuries; sulphonamide crystals; oedema of tubules in acute nephritis. (Renal causes). 3. Obstruction — calculi, strictures, cancer.

Signs and symptoms. Stage 1: *Oliguric phase.* Urinary output markedly reduced — below 30 ml per hour. If overhydration occurs — headache, engorgement of neck veins, full bounding rapid pulse. Blood reveals raised potassium and urea, reduced bicarbonate and haemoglobin. Resistance to infection greatly reduced. Oedema may be marked. This state may persist for several days until kidneys start to regain ability or patient passes into coma and dies. Stage 2: *Diuretic phase.* Gradual increase in urinary output. If overhydration previously, output may be very large — up to 10 litres a day. Severe loss of chloride may cause alkalosis. Urine pale and of low specific gravity due to inability of nephrons to concentrate filtrate. Stage 3: *Recovery phase.* Amount of urine gradually balances intake and power to concentrate returns as new cells grow in nephrons. May be weeks before full function restored.

Treatment in stage 1

Fluid intake restricted to 400 ml plus amount of previous day's output. Careful record of all output kept. Fluids given orally if no vomiting. Failing this, intravenous route used. A fine polythene catheter may be introduced far into a vein so that 40 per cent dextrose can be infused. This method reduces risk of phlebitis and thrombosis when such high concentration of dextrose used. Protein intake reduced to 0:5 g/kg body weight and should consist of first class protein only.

Anaemia can be improved without overloading circulatory system with fluid by giving packed cells 250 ml twice weekly.

Care of skin, mouth and pressure areas must be scrupulous because of high risk of infection. Patients are best isolated with minimum attendants and visitors.

Potassium accumulation may be combatted with ion exchange resins. Resonium A 50 g 8 hourly orally or retention enema 100 g in 120 ml water given at night.

If diuresis does not occur within 5–7 days patient in danger of dying and dialysis may be performed. Indications — potassium raised above 7 mmol, urea raised above 350 mg per cent bicarbonate level below 14 mmol, gross oedema and overhydration.

Dialysis. A means of ridding body of excess water and wastes and correcting electrolyte imbalance. A semipermeable membrane lies between blood and dialysing fluid. The semipermeable membrane may be the peritoneum (peritoneal dialysis) or it may be artifical — a thin tube of polythene or cellophane (artifical kidney, haemodialysis). The semipermeable membrane allows passage of substances from blood into dialysing fluid or the other way round; hence substances in dialysing fluid have to be carefully measured, some to encourage passage of excess substances from blood, others to correct deficiencies in blood. Heparin, added to prevent clotting of blood in haemodialysis, or formation of fibrin in peritoneal dialysis. Antibiotics added to combat risk of infection.

Peritoneal dialysis. Polythene cannula with many small holes in its end, passed through small incision in abdominal wall. Its distal end is placed in the retro-vesicular pouch (pouch of Douglas). Cannula connected to a bottle, or bottles, of dialysing fluid suspended above bed and 2 litres run in rapidly (10 minutes). Fluid allowed to remain in peritoneal space for 10–20 minutes (longer in some cases) and is then drained off and a fresh quantity run in. This may be repeated for days. A careful record of intake and output maintained and returned dialysate sent to laboratory for measurement of its contents. If dialysis continues longer than 48 hours cannula removed and replaced through fresh incision.

Haemodialysis. This is a much more cumbersome procedure requiring special equipment. The semipermeable membrane and tubing leading to and from it must first be filled with compatible blood and must then be linked into the patient's circulatory system. Risks involved are compensated for by rapid correction of accumulated wastes and electrolyte imbalance.

Treatment in stage 2

Dehydration and chloride loss are biggest dangers. Fluid balance charts are even more important and encouragement to take sufficient fluids an important nursing task. Dietary replacement of fluids, chlorides and proteins necessary.

Treatment in stage 3

Supervision of patient with regular checks on kidney function. Albuminuria may persist for many months. Patient should beware of over-exertion and avoid contact with infectious diseases.

Prevention of acute renal failure

Prompt relief of hypotension in shock, haemorrhage, dehydration etc. High fluid intake, orally or intravenously. Forced diuresis — intravenous urea or Mannitol — controlled by actual quantities of urine excreted hourly.

Diseases of the urinary tract: The kidney

Glomerulonephritis

Classification previously hampered by lack of precise information of causes and pathological changes.

Immunofluoroscopy and electron microscopy give more details and allow better understanding of changes. Complexity of structure of glomerulus unravelled and effect of antibodies, antigens, complement fractions studied.

Variety of exogenous and endogenous antigens may form complexes with antibodies which are trapped in glomerular basement membrane between vascular endothelium and Bowmans capsular cells. Complement binds to complexes and attract leucocytes which release enzymes and damage the glomerulus.

Another cause is formation of antibody to basement membrane itself possibly after basement membrane has been altered by drugs, poisons, viruses etc. Similar sequence then occurs — binding of complement, attraction of leukocytes, release of lysosomal enzymes, erosion of surrounding cells with serious alteration of renal function.

Poststreptococcal glomerulonephritis

Classical prototype of exogenous antigen/antibody complex glomerular disruption.

Cause. Recent history of streptococcal infection 10–21 days previously — impetigo, tonsillitis, pharyngitis.

Group A, beta-haemolytic streptococci may be isolated. More often high titre of antistreptolysin (ASO) or antistreptokinose (ASK) or antihyaluronidase (AH) found in serum.

Signs and symptoms. Sudden onset of haematuria, albuminuria, oliguria, hypertension, oedema. Latter causes generalized non-pitting type of oedema noticed first round eyes. Nausea, vomiting, malaise, slight pyrexia, loin pain, convulsions in children.

Diagnosis. Confirmed by high ASO, ASK, and AH, urea, creatinine. Urine shows hyaline and granular casts. Rapid ESR.

Pathology. Proliferation of endothelial and capsular cells which fill and obliterate Bowman's space. Leucocyte infiltration. Oedema of tubule cells. Later, hyalinisation and obliteration of glomeruli.

Treatment. Strict rest in bed until haematuria stops. While oliguria persists (usually 2–5 days) — restrict protein to 0·5 g/kg body weight; restrict fluids to 400 ml plus equivalent of previous day's urinary output; no salt.

Keep careful records of (1) fluid balance, (2) blood pressure, (3) pulse rate, especially sleeping pulse.

Antibiotics — penicillin ½ million units 6 hourly 5–7 days. Benzathene penicillin 750 000 units intramuscularly once a month may be given until the patient is 18–21 years old to prevent further attacks of streptococcal infection.

Complete anuria may occur and need dialysis.

As soon as diuresis sets in, gradually increase fluids, protein and salt according to fluid balance chart.

Prognosis. 1–2 per cent die in initial attack; 5–10 per cent recover incompletely and continue to have albuminuria and hypertension; remainder recover completely.

Complications. Urinary infection. Renal failure. Hypertensive encephalopathy (fits, coma). Chronic nephritis. Carditis and congestive cardiac failure.

Prevention. Contacts of patients who suffer streptococcal infections should have throat swabs taken and any revealing beta haemolytic streptococci should have one injection of benzathene penicillin 600 000 units.

Nephrotic syndrome

Nephritis with an insidious onset characterized by albuminuria, oedema, low blood albumin, lipiduria, hyperlipdaemia.

Cause. Unknown. May arise in course of diabetes mellitus, malaria, congestive heart failure and constrictive paricarditis. May follow chilling and exposure.

Classification. Depends on electron microscopy and immuno-fluorescent studies on biopsy material; (a) Only minimal lesion disease. Swelling of basement membrane and disordered podocytes seen. No antibody/antigen/complement deposition. (b) Membranous disease. No cellular proliferation. Swelling of capillary endothelium. Lumpy deposits of immunoglobulins and complement between endothelium and basement membrane. (c) Proliferative disease. Mesangial proliferation and obliteration of glomeruli. Complement deposition but not immunoglobulin.

Signs and symptoms. Gradual increase of oedema over 2–3 weeks, swelling round ankles first, increasing to generalized severe oedema with peritoneal, and sometimes pleural and pericardial effusion. Oliguria while oedema is developing. Malaise and anorexia may be severe. Muscle wasting usually hidden by oedema. Intercurrent infections may be severe — upper respiratory tract, skin, gastro-intestinal tract. Urine shows albumin, granular casts. Blood examination shows diminished albumin and high cholesterol level.

Treatment. Nil specific. Rest in bed while oedema severe. Keep warm. Avoid chills. Fluids given to allay thirst but no attempt to 'push' fluids. Salt restricted — none added to meals: may be sufficient, but if oedema severe may be necessary to omit from cooking as well. Measures to reduce oedema include acupuncture, insertion of Southey's tubes, paracentesis of abdomen and thorax.

Observations and charts include: daily estimation of urinary albumin, preferably from a 24 hour rather than a single specimen; daily weight chart; measurement of abdominal girth; daily blood pressure. Blood taken weekly for levels of protein, cholesterol, urea, sodium, potassium, chlorides, and bicarbonates. Urea clearance test gives good guide to renal function.

Diuretics to encourage salt excretion may be given. Chlorothiazide 1–2 g daily together with potassium chloride to prevent potassium depletion. Frusemide. Ethacrynic acid. Spironolactone. Mercurials avoided.

Steroids usually given in high dosage. Prednisolone 2 mg/kg/day up to 100 mg for 10 days then tailed off over 30 days followed by ACTH 10–20 units twice weekly for 2 weeks. If oedema returns or if albuminuria persists, a second course may be given. Intermittent courses — 20–50 mg 4 days a week may be given until one month after cessation of albuminuria. Dose tailed off by halving it at monthly intervals until it is reduced to 10 mg. Milk or calcium gluconate given to lessen decalcification of bones with such long courses of steroids.

Infections treated promptly with appropriate antibiotics.

Prognosis. Adults do poorly: 50 per cent die within three years of onset. Children: 60 per cent — 90 per cent recover with modern treatment. High proportion develop chronic renal failure and uraemia.

Complications. Malignant hypertension. Congestive cardiac failure. Respiratory infections. Renal tract infection.

Chronic renal insufficiency

Gradually increasing loss of nephrons and inability to maintain optimum blood levels of water, salts electrolytes, acids and bases.

Causes. Glomerulonephritis. Secondary to other diseases — diabetes mellitus, gout, pericarditis, congestive cardiac failure. Poisons — troxidone, phenytoin (in treatment of epilepsy), mercurials, gold.

Pathology. Depends on cause. Typical changes found following acute glomerulonephritis — hyalinized glomeruli, tubules obliterated, others hypertrophied; diabetes — focal deposits of intercapillary sclerosis; hypertension — 'onion-skin' glomeruli; amyloid disease — deposits of clear jelly-like material round small vessels; polycystic disease — blind ally nephrons, etc.

In all, a gradual reduction in functional tissue causing gradual reduction in kidney's ability to maintain excretion of wastes, fluid and electrolyte balance, production of haemopoetic factors.

Stages. (1) Latent stage. Few symptoms apart from constant loss of albumin in urine. (2) Oedematous stage. (3) Uraemic stage.

Signs and symptoms. Latent stage: Variable length, occasionally several years. Transient oedema of ankles. Hypertension 150–180 systolic. Occasional severe haedaches. Patient tires easily. Albuminuria. Anaemia. Oedematous stage. Marked generalized oedema. Muscle wasting. Malaise. Anorexia. Hypertension. Intercurrent infections common. Uraemic stage: Headache. Nausea. Vomiting. Hiccough. Dyspnoea. Muscle twitching leading to convulsions and coma. Uraemic 'frost' on skin. Musty odour to sweat and breath.

Treatment. Latent stage: Lead as full a life as possible without fatigue or exhaustion. As much rest as possible without actually becoming a voluntary invalid. Avoid chills. Treat all infections promptly and thoroughly, especially urinary tract infections. High protein diet: 150–200 g daily — in an attempt to keep blood albumin up to normal and delay onset of oedematous stage. Oedematous stage: Treat oedema with chlorothiazide diuretics, acupuncture, Southey's tubes, paracentesis. Treat hypertension. Venepuncture and rapid removal of 500 ml blood may give relief. Uraemic stage: Reduce fluids. Exclude salt. Low protein diet until diuresis occurs. Salt may be used in cooking thereafter. Dialysis may be necessary. Sedatives to control twitching. Light anaesthesia for convulsions.

Prognosis. Fatal termination but patient may be kept active and alert till the end, especially if only first class proteins are given for low protein diet. Eggs with added methionine form the basis of this type of diet. Renal transplantation offers hope in selected cases.

Hydronephrosis

Dilatation of pelvis of kidney with retained urine which may progress to destruction of kidney substance.

Causes. Partial obstruction of free flow of urine into bladder — calculus, neoplasm of wall of ureter, pressure on ureter from outside, e.g. ovarian cyst, kinking of ureter due to mobile kidney.

Signs and symptoms. Usually vague. Aching pain in loin with occasional bouts of renal colic. May be palpable mass in loin. If retained urine becomes infected — pyrexia, nausea, vomiting, malaise, anorexia.

Treatment. Surgical correction of partial obstruction to prevent destruction of renal tissue. Nephrectomy thereafter.

Renal calculi

Development of stones precipitated out of urine. Occur in calices or in pelvis of kidney.

Cause. One renal function is to concentrate urine by reabsorbing water from glomerular filtrate. This may create a saturated solution of calcium salts some of which are thrown out of solution. Infected material, casts and blood clots encourage deposition of calcium by forming a nucleus upon which stone is built. Other factors — hyperparathyroidism with higher blood levels of calcium; stasis of patients confined to bed especially in recumbent position.

Types of calculus. Usually mixed but often one substance predominates — calcium oxalate, calcium phosphate, calcium carbonate, ammonium magnesium phosphate. More rarely — uric acid, cystine, xanthine.

Signs and symptoms. May be none when stone remains in kidney pelvis and does not cause obstruction. If partial obstruction occurs — hydronephrosis (see p. 118). If stone dislodges — acute attack of renal colic — severe pain starting in loin and shooting round into abdomen and down into thigh, scrotum or groin. Pain causes shock — pallor, sweating, low blood pressure, nausea and vomiting. May cause haematuria.

Stones containing calcium are radio-opaque.

Treatment of colic. Pethidine 100 mg and atropine 0.6 mg or metochlopramide (Maxolon) 10 mg I.M. Apply warmth to loin. Hot bath. Sudden cold to loin may stop pain — ethyl chloride sprayed from distance of 12 inches for 3–4 seconds. If stone lodges in ureter surgical removal necessary. Stone may remain in bladder and cause pain especially at end of micturition, or it may be passed via urethra.

Prevention of stone formation. High fluid intake especially before retiring, even if this means having to wake during night to pass urine. Avoidance of milk and milk products. Frequent turning of bed ridden patients. Prompt treatment of urinary tract infections.

Nephrocalcinosis

Definition. Deposition of calcium salts throughout renal substance. (Sometimes combined with stone formation).

Cause. High serum calcium, or phosphate due to high calcium intake especially if combined with high vitamin D intake (food freaks), hyperparathyroidism, chronic pyelonephritis, immobilization in bed, sarcoidois.

Signs and symptoms. May be asymptomatic. Anaemia, chronic renal insufficiency, X-ray shows minute scattered opacities.

Treatment. High fluid intake. Treat cause.

Prognosis. If cause treated vigorously progress slowed down but renal insufficiency generally progressive.

Analgesic nephropathy

Definition. Acute papillary necrosis associated with chronic ingestion of aspirin/phenacetin combinations for chronic headache, 'rheumatism', or just to achieve a lift in mood.

Signs and symptoms. Typically middle-aged female with haematuria, polyuria, anaemia, frequent urinary tract infections, raised blood urea and creatinine.

Diagnosis. IVP shows clubbing of calices.

Treatment. As for chronic renal insufficiency.

Movable kidney

Mobility of kidney greater than normal. Kidney may descend causing kinking of ureter.

Incidence. Females more than males (10:1). Common age 30–40 years.

Contributory factors. Loss of perinephric fat. Loss of tone of abdominal muscles and visceroptosis.

Signs and symptoms. May be none — discovered accidentally at general examination. May be slight — dragging ache in loin. May be severe — renal colic, tenderness in loin, oliguria until lying flat and then passage of large quantity of urine with cessation of pain.

Diagnosis. Confirmed by pyelography.

Treatment. (1) Encourage increase in fat deposits with high calorie diet. Increase tone of abdominal muscles with suitable exercises. (2) Surgical — fixation of kidney (nephropexy). Nephrectomy if hydronephrosis has progressed too far.

Pyelitis

Inflammation of kidney pelvis.

Cause. Usually infection with *E. coli* (colon bacillus) or *B. proteus*. Occasionally staphylococcal or streptococcal infection.

Spread of organisms. (1) Via blood stream, e.g. from endocarditis. (2) Up urinary tract from bladder.

Contributory factors. Stasis of urine and partial obstruction — calculi, prostatomegaly, neurogenic spasm of urethral sphincter; pregnancy and compression of ureters against pelvic brim; previous infection; diabetes; catheterization.

Danger. Spread of infection to kidney substance — pyelonephritis.

Signs and symptoms. Sudden pyrexia with rigors. Pain and tenderness in loin. Renal colic as pus passes down ureter. Frequency due to irritation of trigone. Scalding sensation of micturition due to inflammation of urethra.

Treatment. Complete rest in bed while pyrexia persists. Large fluid intake — 3 litres per day (ingenuity of nursing staff may be taxed to get patient to drink so much, encourage by conscientious visits every 15 minutes and offering as much variety of fluids as possible). Urinary antiseptics according to sensitivity of organism — sulphonamides, nitrofurantoin, antibiotics.

Neoplasm of kidney

Types. Carcinoma — rare. Sarcoma — rare. Blastocytoma (Wilms' tumour) embryonic tissue present, rapid growth with metastases — rare but accounts for ⅓ of kidney tumours in children. Adenosarcoma — may be encapsulated in early stages but grows rapidly and metastasises to lungs and bones.

Signs and symptoms. Haematuria. Rapid wasting. Pain variable. Palpable mass in flank. Varicocele may occur due to obstruction of spermatic vein.

Diagnosis. Confirmed by intravenous urography.

Treatment. Nephrectomy and ureterectomy followed by deep X-ray therapy.

Prognosis. Very poor.

Tuberculosis of kidney

Tubercular infection almost always secondary to pulmonary tuberculosis.

Cause. Spread of organism via blood into one kidney. Other kidney may be infected similarly or infection may travel to bladder and then up ureter.

Signs and symptoms. Frequency. Haematuria. Pyuria.

Diagnosis. Cystoscopy may reveal pus issuing from ureter. Guinea-pig inoculation with centrifuge deposit from 24 hour specimen of urine. Pyelography may show abnormal shape of calices or pelvis.

Treatment. Responds rapidly to antitubercular drugs.

Complications. Spread of tuberculosis to ureters, bladder, prostrate, vas deferens, epididymis, testes.

Congenital abnormalities

1. Unilateral kidney. One kidney fails to develop. No symptoms. Importance — condition relatively common hence need for full investigation when surgery of remaining kidney contemplated.

2. *Double kidney*. Common. Results from imperfect development for segmental origin in foetus. Usually double pelvis and often double ureter. Often one pelvis or ureter is imperfect and causes hydronephrosis. Treatment — surgical (partial nephrectomy).

3. *Miniature kidney*. One kidney fails to reach full size but is often a perfect functioning miniature. The number of nephrons it contains may be insufficient to support life if other kidney has to be removed.

4. *Horseshoe kidney*. Kidneys are united at their lower poles in front of vertebral column. Often their blood supply is abnormal being derived from lower aorta or from internal iliac arteries. Usually they function normally but there is an increased risk of infection and hydronephrosis.

5. *Ectopic kidney*. During development, kidneys form in pelvis and ascend to their final position high in abdominal cavity. Sometimes their ascent is interrupted and one of them comes to rest against the sacrum, or pelvic brim, or iliac fossa. Often such kidneys are poorly developed and prone to infection, calculi formation and hydronephrosis.

6. *Additional renal arteries*. These arise directly from aorta and may enter kidney via hilum or directly into upper or lower pole. Common (1 in 5 of population). Usually sole blood supply to a section of kidney and damage to them results in renal infarction.

7. *Polycystic kidney*. During development collecting tubules grown inwards to meet outward growing nephrons. If they fail to meet, a cystic kidney develops. (Other congenital abnormalities may exist — cysts of liver, pancreas, ovaries; abnormally low ears). Most cases die shortly after birth. Minor degrees may permit life without symptoms until about 40 years of age, then, pain, haematuria or symptoms of chronic renal failure — hypertension, uraemia. No curative treatment. Urinary infections should be treated promptly. Sudden severe pain may be treated by puncturing and draining larger cysts. Recently life prolonged by kidney transplant.

The ureters

Congenital abnormalities

1. Double ureter. Not uncommon. May be complete and enter bladder independently. Often joins other ureter. Usually free of symptoms. Occasionally causes hydronephrosis because of urinary reflux from one ureter back up the other.

2. Mega ureter. Ureter dilated and holds urine which becomes infected. Cause not known.

3. Ureterocele. Projection of lower end of ureter into bladder forming cyst-like sac. May become large enough to fill bladder. Treatment is to excise sac and repair ureteric orifice.

The bladder

Congenital abnormalities

1. Ectopic bladder. Multiple deformity — absence of pubic rami and skin over pubic area, abnormal urethra, cleft clitoris, absence of anterior bladder wall with exposure of its interior. Infection occurs readily. Closure may be attempted but incontinence remains. Transplantation of ureters into colon occasionally successful.

2. Congenital vesicular diverticulum. Usually due to obstruction of urethral opening.

Nocturnal enuresis

Involuntary micturition during sleep. Usually in children but may persist into adult life.

Cause. Usually psychological but organic causes should be excluded — polyuria from diabetes, urinary infection, faulty sphincter.

Treatment. Limit fluid intake after 4 p.m. Installation of electric alarm system which ring a bell and wakes patient is soon as micturition starts to wet a pad — sometimes successful. Most cases clear spontaneously at or soon after puberty. Tricyclic antidepressants, e.g. Toframil up to 100 mg nightly effective in many cases.

Retention of urine

Bladder full but patient unable to pass urine.

Causes. (1) Congenital. Hypertrophy of internal sphincter;

stenosis of urethra; valvular mucosa of urethra. (2) Obstruction. Calculus lodged in urethra; urethritis; prostatitis; prostatomegaly; cancer. (3) Pressure from outside urethra — carcinoma of vulva, loaded rectum in children. (4) Neurogenic. Inability of sphincter to relax — after low abdominal and pelvic surgery, haemorrhoidectomy, spinal injury, hysteria.

Types. (1) Acute, (2) Chronic.

Acute retention. Sudden obstruction causing painful distension of bladder which must be relieved without delay — catheteriztion, suprapubic puncture, surrapubic cystotomy.

Treatment. Postoperative neurogenic retention may be relieved with carbachol 0·25 mg subcutaneously.

Hysterical neurogenic retention may be relieved with simple remedies — stand male patient erect, leave in privacy, sound of splashing water or running tap, sit female patient on warm bedpan containing hot water.

If indwelling catheter has to be inserted it should be of nonirritating latex or plastic and connected immediately to underwater seal drainage bottle containing antiseptic.

Chronic retention. Partial obstruction, Incomplete emptying of bladder. Slow distension and painless dilatation of bladder. Bladder becomes atonic and full of urine which readily becomes infected. May be constant dribbling of urine — retention with overflow. Preceded by frequency, hesitancy, poor stream. Acute retention may supervene. Danger — chronic kidney failure.

Treatment. Investigate degree of kidney damage — blood urea, electrolyte imbalance, anaemia. Catheter drainage or suprapubic cystotomy to allow time for correction of blood urea, low haemoglobin, urinary infection and eletrolyte imbalance.

Extreme care must be taken to prevent further infection — catheterization under strict aseptic precautions, immediate connection to under-water seal bottle containing antiseptic, or disposable bag. Careful cleansing of urethral meatus twice daily and application of antiseptic cream.

When blood chemistry has been corrected or stabilized, surgical correction of obstruction attempted.

Neoplasm of bladder

Most cases are carcinoma arising from epithelial cells.

Aetiology. Usually over 60 years. Males more commonly than females (3:1). (Occupational hazard among dye workers. The carcinogenic agents are naphthylamine and bezidine. Onset 18 years after start in dye works).

Types. Papilloma, carcinoma, epithelioma, adenocarcinoma.

Signs and symptoms. Painless haematuria — fresh bright blood or clots. Later — frequency and pain. Very late — palpable mass above pubis or on rectal or vaginal examination.

Diagnosis. Confirmed by cystoscopy, biopsy and urography.

Treatment. Surgical removal of either tumour or part of bladder or whole bladder with transplantation of ureters. Palliative measure only — transplantation of ureters to prevent painful frequency. Irradiation with radon seeds or deep X-ray therapy.

Diverticulum of bladder

Pouch-like outgrowth from wall of bladder.

Cause. Partial obstruction of urinary outflow causing residual urine and atony of bladder wall.

Diagnosis. Urography. Cystoscopy.

Signs and symptoms. Mostly those of urinary obstruction — prostatomegaly, urethral stricture, cystitis and chronic renal failure. Urine becomes infected readily and is resistant to urinary antiseptics.

Treatment. Primarily — remove or correct cause of obstruction. Single diverticulum — excised. Multiple diverticulae excision of bladder and transplantation of ureters.

Complications. Fistulae connecting with vagina or rectum.

Cystitis

Inflammation of bladder.

Causes. Infection descending from kidney or ascending from urethra. Catheterization can introduce organisms.

Predisposing factors. Stasis of urine and existing bladder conditions — cancer, diverticula, calculi, fistula.

Types. (1) Acute; (2) confined to trigone; (3) chronic; (4) Hunner's ulceration.

Acute. Signs and symptoms. Sudden onset with urgency, frequency, suprapubic pain, scalding pain on micturition and pain in tip of penis after micturition. Urine cloudy, may be streaked with blood passed after main stream of urine. Offensive odour. May be rigor at onset followed by mild pyrexia.

Diagnosis. Confirmed by microscopic examination of centrifuge deposit of urine for pus cells. Culture for organisms and sensitivity.

Treatment. Cause of cystitis sought and treated. Rest in bed while pyrexia persists — usually 2–3 days. Keep warm. Hot water bottle to lower abdomen a great comfort. Broad spectrum antibiotics or nitrofurantoin (Furadantin) may be given pending sensitivity report. Antispasmodic if urgency becomes intolerable — propanthine bromide. Streptomycin effective in most urinary infections 0·5 g twice daily 4–6 days. More effective if urine is alkaline hence, potassium citrate 1–2 g 4 hourly.

Trigonitis. (Trigone — triangular area between ureteric and urethral orifices where bladder is attached to floor of pelvis). Often the only inflamed area in descending infections from pyelitis and pyelonephritis. More common in women.

Signs and symptoms. As for cystitis.

Treatment. Often resistant to treatment. Nitrofurantoin for several weeks after symptoms abate to prevent recurrence. Fibrosis and polyposis of urethral orifice may cause chronic obstruction and need surgical repair.

Chronic. Occurs in bladder conditions where surgical correction may not be possible — cancer, fistula.

Signs and symptoms. Frequency. Infected urine.

Treatment. Long course of antibiotics to which organisms are sensitive. Continuous bladder irrigation. High fluid intake. Encourage micturition at regular fixed intervals.

Hunner's ulceration. Chronic cystitis with ulceration.

Cause. Unknown.

Aetiology. Women between 50 and 60 years.

Pathology. Isolated patches of inflammation which bleed readily and leave ulcers.

Signs and symptoms. Suprapubic pain may be severe. Frequency, urgency, (especially at night), haematuria. Urine sterile. Tends to clear spontaneously but fibrotic contraction of bladder may occur — patient unable to retain more than 60–100 ml urine.

Treatment. Diathermy of ulcers via cystoscope. Corticosteroid therapy to reduce inflammation. Prevention of contracture by distension of the bladder under general anaesthetic. If contracture has occurred — colocystoplasty (segment of colon isolated, split open and used as a patch, still attached to its mesentery, to replace the ulcerated section of bladder wall).

The urethra

Congenital abnormalities

1. Hypospadias. Urethra opens somewhere under penis instead of running a course to its tip. Absence of corpus spongiosum gives rise to fibrotic shortening of penis and inability to erect penis without causing a painful downward curvature (chordee). Lesser degress occur with urethral meatus situated an inch or so from tip. Attempts made to reconstruct urethra by skin grafting.

2. Epispadias. Displacement of urethra to upper surface of penis where it runs as a gutter instead of an enclosed tube. In the most severe form, sphincters are incomplete and incontinence occurs. Often associated with ectopic bladder. Treatment: suprapubic cystotomy to divert urine while a false urethral tube is formed by skin grafting (at about 4–6 years old).

The penis

Phimosis

Stenosis or narrowing of orifice of prepuce so that it cannot be pulled back over the glans.

Signs and symptoms. Usually none but predisposes to balanitis.

Treatment. Some degree of adherence of prepuce to glans is common at birth and needs no treatment unless it is obstructing urethral meatus, then, gentle tension is usually enough to break down the adhesions sufficiently to allow free flow of urine. Circumcision may be performed.

Paraphimosis

Inability to draw prepuce forward over glans after erection of penis. Constricting band of prepuce causes oedema of glans and of prepuce itself and, if untreated, may become gangrenous.

Treatment. Reduction under general anaesthesia. Dorsal slit. Injection of hyalase to disperse oedema.

Priapism

Painful erection of penis without sexual stimulation or desire.

Causes. Thrombosis of veins draining corpora cavernosa. May follow circumcision (without thrombosis). May occur in paraplegia.

Treatment. Morphia given for pain. Catheterisation necessary but extreme pain necessitates general anaesthetic for insertion of catheter. Anticoagulant therapy. If ineffective — incision of corpora cavernosa and evacuation of clots. Amputation of penis if gangrene threatens.

In priapism without thrombosis — application of cold compresses, bromides e.g. potassium bromide 0·5–1 g at night, stilboestrol 5 mg thrice daily 2–3 days.

Balanitis
Inflammation of glans penis.

Cause. Usually secondary infection of accumulated smegma (odoriferous cheesy excretion from glands in the glans penis). May occur in association with cancer of penis.

Signs and symptoms. Pain and oedema of glans and prepuce.

Treatment. Retraction of prepuce. Careful and gentle cleaning with cetrimide followed by application of chlorhexidine cream.

Neoplasm of penis
Epithelioma. Almost unknown among races which practise ritual circumcision.

Cause. Possible chronic irritation from balanitis.

Signs and symptoms. Painless wart-like mass with offensive bloodstained purulent discharge. Slowly progressive.

Treatment. Radium mould fitted round penis and applied for carefully timed periods each day. If diagnosed early — partial amputation. In advanced cases — total amputation plus scrotum, testes and inguinal glands.

Orchitis
Inflammation of testis.

Causes. Viraemia (mumps); bacillaemia (typhoid); direct spread of organisms via vas deferens following prostatic surgery; occasionally tuberculosis or syphilis.

Signs and symptoms. Pain, redness, heat swelling, tenderness, pyrexia.

Treatment. Elevate scrotum on elastoplast bridge between thighs. Rest in bed while pyrexia persists. Appropriate antibiotics.

Epididymitis

Inflammation of epididymis (fine coiled tube attached to posterior border of testis in which spermatozoa are stored pending discharge via vas deferens).

Causes. Bacterial spread from bladder or urethra. Often associated with urinary infections. More common after prostatectomy. May be blood-borne — tuberculosis, syphilis.

Signs and symptoms. Pain, redness and swelling of scrotum. Tenderness severe. Mass palpable adjacent to testis.

Treatment. Rest in bed with scrotal support. Analgesics. Antibiotics.

Complications. Breakdown of skin over epididymis and exposure of scrotal contents. Sterility.

Hydrocele

Collection of sterile fluid within the tunica vaginalis (double fold of peritoneum surrounding the testis).

Cause. Unknown.

Signs and symptoms. Swelling of scrotum on one side. Painless.

Treatment. Aspirations when swelling reaches embarrassing proportions. Excision of tunica vaginalis cures.

The prostate

Prostatomegaly

Benign enlargement of prostate gland. Some enlargement is common in most men after 50 years.

Cause. Unknown. Possibly hormone imbalance.

Signs and symptoms. Very variable. Sometimes none even with considerable enlargement. Usually increasing difficulty in passing urine, poor stream, residual urine. If urine becomes infected — pyrexia, urgency, frequency.

Complications. Pyelitis and pyelonephritis. If residual urine is large — retention with overflow (constant, dribbling incontinence), chronic renal failure, uraemia.

Diagnosis. Confirmed by rectal examination, cystoscopy.

Treatment. Depends on several factors — age, physical state, mental state, existence of concurrent diseases such as cardiac or respiratory failure.

Surgical removal if patient considered fit, if sudden acute

retention occurs, if there are signs of renal failure, or if reinfections occurs constantly.

Diuretics: Drugs which increase urinary secretion

Mode of action

1. Antagonises enzymes engaged in reabsorption — mercurials.

2. Enhances excretion of sodium and/or potassium salts thus raising osmotic pressure of filtrate in tubules — chlorothiazides.

3. Increases osmotic force of filtrate by supplying additional solutes — urea, salines, e.g. potassium citrate, sodium citrate.

4. Increases permeability of glomerular capillaries, thus allowing increased escape of filtrate — caffeine, theobromine, theophylline.

5. Inhibits action of hormone aldosterone which reabsorbs sodium. Increased sodium in filtrate raises its osmotic pressure and encourages retention of water in filtrate — spironolactone (Aldactone A).

6. Antagonises action of anti-diuretic hormone — bromaleate (neo Bromth).

7. Encourages secretion of solutes into filtrate by inhibiting action of carbonic anhydrase — acetazolamide (Diamox).

8. Reduces damage and swelling of glomerular capillaries by lowering blood pressure — antihypertensive drugs e.g. rauwolfia, reserpine.

9. Improving general circulation — cardiac diuretics e.g. digitalis, quinidine, aminophylline, apresoline.

Common diuretics

1. Mercurials

Mersalyl, Mercuhydrin, Mercuprocyl, Thiomerin.

Administration. Usual route — intramuscular injection. May be given intravenously if immediate action desired. Oral route possible but degree of absorption uncertain.

Occasional idiosyncrasy found — test dose 0·5 ml and observe for ½ hour — pain in abdomen, nausea, vomiting, vertigo, pyrexia. If none occur, dosage: 1 to 2 ml — alternate days until body weight and fluid balance stabilises, then once or twice weekly to keep free from oedema.

Indications. Congestive cardiac failure. Cardiac oedema. Ascites. Anasarca. Nephrosis. Selected cases of subacute and chronic nephritis.

Contra-indications. Acute nephritis, Idiosyncrasy. Acute renal failure.

Side effects. Excessive diuresis and dehydration. Electrolyte imbalance due to excessive sodium and potassium loss — muscle weakness, exhaustion, cramps, acidosis.

2(a) *Thiazide and its compounds*

Chlorothiazide, methyclothiazide, hydrochlorothiazide, benthiazide, quinethazone, trichlormethiazide, bendrofuazide, hydroflumenthiazide, polythiazide. (Many trade names — Chlotride, Enduron, Esidrex, Exna, Hydromox, Aprinox, Saluron, Renese).

Administration. Oral tablets. 0·5 to 2 g daily in divided doses. To prevent uncomfortable nocturia doses should cease by mid-afternoon.

Indications. Oedema from any cause — cardiac, renal, hepatic, premenstrual, pregnancy, steroid induced, obesity (fluid retention phase).

Side effects. Rare — potassium depletion (citrus fruits or supplemental potassium citrate may prevent this).

Potentiates action of other drugs, especially antihypertensives and digitalis. Patients *must* be closely observed to prevent overdosage of these.

2(b) *Furosemide (Lasix) and Ethacrynic acid (Edecril)*

Very powerful. Act like thiazides by inhibiting reabsorption of sodium from tubules. Rapid action of short duration. May be given i.v., i.m. or orally. May cause severe hyponatraemia and hypopotassaemia.

3. *Saline diuretics*

Moderately effective diuretics.

Administration. Oral solutions. Potassium nitrate 0·3–1 g; potassium citrate 1–2 g; potassium sulphate 2–16 g; ammonium chloride 3–6 g.

Side effects. Irritation of gastro-intestinal mucosa — nausea, vomiting, diarrhoea. In patients with renal failure potassium is not readily excreted and blood levels may reach dangerous levels.

4. Acetazolamide (Diamox)

Carbonic anhydrase inhibitor.

Administration. Oral tablets. 0·25–1 g daily. Rapidly absorbed and excreted. Diuresis completed by evening if morning dose given.

Side effects. Drowsiness, numbness in fingers and lips, loss of muscle tone. Agranulocytosis — very rare.

5. Aldosterone inhibitor

Spironolactone (Aldactone A).

Administration. Oral tablets. 25 mg 4 times daily. Should be given in conjunction with other diuretics — usually mercurial or thiazide — when it enhances their effects. Onset of diuresis with spironolactone is delayed — 2 to 3 days. Courses last 2–3 weeks and therapy continued with conventional diuretics alone.

Side effects. Potassium retention which may be serious if patient already has a high blood potassium. Drowsiness and mental confusion. Gynaecosmastia — rare.

6. Digitalis

Other cardiac stimulators produce a diuresis when given to patients with circulatory insufficiency. No such effect in normal persons.

5. The Endocrine System

Pituitary gland (Hypophysis): Disorders of anterior pituitary secretion (adenohypophysis)

Gigantism

General overgrowth of all tissue and organs occurring before closure of epiphyseal cartilages.

Cause. Oversecretion of growth hormone during childhood. Usually due to adenoma.

Signs and symptoms. General overgrowth, before age 15 and over 6 feet tall. Body well proportioned. Strong, alert and intelligent with gentle disposition.

Diagnosis. Direct measurement of plasma growth hormone. In normal persons growth hormone level is high in fasting state and falls to less than 1 ng/ml within 2 hours of oral glucose load.

In gigantism and acromegaly response to glucose load is absent.

X-ray of pituitary fossa may show alteration in shape and size. Examination of visual fields to exclude pressure on optic chiasma. Other hormones may be secondarily affected — Thyroxine, insulin.

Treatment Bromocriptine (Parlodel) reduces growth hormone secretion. May be used alone in mild cases.

Deep X-ray therapy, alpha particle radiation therapy, gland destruction by surgical removal or by yttrium implantation are all effective forms of treatment.

Complications. Optic nerve pressure. Hypopituitarism later-gland becomes exhausted.

Acromegaly

Overgrowth of certain parts of body occurring after closure of epiphyseal cartilages.

Cause. Oversecretion of growth hormone due to adenoma.

Signs and symptoms. Increasing size of head, hands and feet. Bones affected: flat bones of cranium, mandible, phalanges. Enlargement of mandible may interfere with mastication. Organic overgrowth includes, tongue, lips, skin and all internal organs. Psychiatric disturbance common — emotional instability, unreasonable behaviour, depression, persecution complex.

Diagnosis. Typical appearance. X-ray may reveal adenoma. Visual field disturbance.

Treatment. As in gigantism.

Complications. Pressure on optic chiasma with visual field disturbance and eventual blindness. Goitre and raised metabolic rate but rarely hyperthyroidism. Mild diabetes with resistance to insulin. Loss of sexual desire (libido) and atrophy of gonads. Sterility. Osteoarthritis. Pituitary insufficiency develops from exhaustion of gland.

Dwarfism

Failure to grow to full stature. Many degrees of pituitary dwarfism. Absolute lack of growth hormone rare.

Cause. Congenital lack of growth hormone.

Signs and symptoms. Perfectly proportioned individual of small stature. Mentality unimpaired. Pale yellow skin. Slow sexual maturation, occasionally complete sexual failure.

Treatment. Epiphyseal cartilages may remain unossified long after they normally close (due to diminished or absent sex hormones) and growth may be stimulated by administration of growth hormone.

Complications. Blindness due to pressure on optic chiasma. Obesity. Sterility.

Panhypopituitarism

Post-pubertal reduction of all anterior lobe hormones characterized by atrophy and diminished output of target endocrine glands for trophic hormones — thyroid, adrenals, gonads.

Cause. (1) Adenoma of pituitary gland. (2) Post-partum thrombosis of hypothalamic-hypophyseal portal circulation. (3) 'Burning out' of glandular cells following prolonged oversecretion. (4) Brain injury. (5) Craniopharyngioma. (6) Hypophysectomy.

Signs and symptoms. Depends on pattern of hormone deficiency. Atrophy of thyroid gland leading to myxoedema. Atrophy of gonads leading to loss of libido, sterility, amenorrhoea, loss of pubic and axillary hair.

Atrophy of adrenal glands leading to Addison's disease (p. 154). Extreme loss of weight. Muscle weakness. Sensitivity to cold.

Diagnosis. Recent improvement of techniques allow accurate measurement of hormone levels. Confirmed by detecting absence of hormones from thyroid, gonads and adrenal glands. Low plasma protein-bound iodine (PBI). Low uptake of radioactive iodine by thyroid gland (RAI). Lowered metabolic rate (BMR). Low urinary hydrocortisone and gonadotrophin. Normochromic anaemia. Extreme sensitivity to insulin. X-ray of skull may show tumour or abnormality of pituitary fossa.

Treatment. Removal of gland followed by hormone replacement. Ideally this would consist of stimulating the thyroid, adrenal and gonad glands with their respective trophic hormones. Unfortunately TSH and ACTH need to be injected daily and gonodotrophins set up an immunological response in time. Hence, treatment consists of giving thyroxine, cortisone, testosterone and oestrogens. Cortisone 5 mg daily increasing to 30 mg. Testosterone cyclopentyl proprionate 100–200 mg every 3–4 weeks.

Complications. Water intoxication following excess fluid intake due to cortisone which limits rate of excretion of water. Excessive appetite and obesity also due to cortisone. Addisonian crisis if thyroid extract given in too large a quantity before instituting cortisone therapy.

Hyperprolactinaemia

Oversecretion of prolactin.

Causes Pituitary tumours. Hypothalamic disorder causing reduction in prolactin-inhibiting factor.

Hypothyroidism.

Secondary to some drugs — phenothiazines, metochlopramide, methyl dopa, cimetidine, MOA inhibitors.

Signs and symptoms. In women — amenorrhoea, infertility, galactorrhoea.

In men — testicular atrophy, sterility, gynaecomastia, galactorrhoea.

Treatment. Removal of pituitary tumour. Correction of other causes. Bromocriptine 2·5 mg t.i.d. restores gonadotrophins secretion if pituitary is normal.

Froehlich's syndrome

Obesity and genital atrophy.

Cause. Anterior pituitary insufficiency secondary to hypothalamic disorder.

Signs and symptoms. General adiposity. Underdevelopment of secondary sexual characteristics and sexual organs. Occasionally mental retardation, lethargy and knock-knees.

Treatment. If presence of tumour can be established — deep X-ray therapy.

Cushing's syndrome

Primarily a disease of the adrenal glands. Occasionally the oversecretion of cortical hormones is due to an oversection of ACTH. Such patients often have deep pigmentation of skin.

Treatment. Extirpation of pituitary gland by deep X-ray therapy or hypophysectomy.

Disorders of posterior pituitary secretion (Neurohypophysis)

Oxytocin insufficiency

Oxytocin production normally increases during last days of pregnancy. When this fails to occur, labour is prolonged and uterine contractions poor. Oxytocin also produced in response to babe suckling and causes release of accumulated milk into alveoli leading to nipples. Insufficiency of oxytocin causes retention of milk which inhibits production of lactogenic hormone (luteotrophin, prolactin), thus milk production ceases. While lactogenic hormone is being produced, follicle stimulating hormone and lueteinising hormone is suppressed, so that ovulation and menstruation do not occur.

Diabetes insipidus

Passage of large quantities of pale urine containing few solutes and hence of low specific gravity. Intense unquenchable thirst (polydipsia).

Cause. Defect in chain of events leading to release of antidiuretic hormone (ADH) from posterior pituitary. ADH secreted in hypothalamus, conveyed to posterior pituitary and released on receipt of impulses from special centres in hypothalamus which are sensitive to concentration of solutes in blood (osmolality). Injury to these centres is the prime cause of diabetes insipidus — trauma, tumours, meningitis, cerebrovascular accident.

Signs and symptoms. Passage of large amounts of pale urine, 10–20 litres per day. Specific gravity below 1005. Insatiable thirst (stopping drinking does not stop the polyuria). Severe dehydration occurs rapidly if patient unable to drink — if unconscious, anaesthetized etc.

Diagnosis. Condition easy to diagnose. Cause may be difficult to trace. Hickey-Hare test — intravenous infusion of hypertonic saline causes increase in urinary output; administration of 0·2–0·3 ml of ADH decreases output. Exhaustive tests to find cause — lumbar puncture, X-ray of skull and chest for metastatic cancer, Wassermann and Kahn for syphilis, marrow biopsy for multiple myeloma.

Treatment. Correction of underlying cause if possible. Specific treatment — intramuscular injection of vasopressin tannate in oil 0·5–1 ml. Effect is immediate and lasts 24–72 hours. (Active ingredient tends to settle as thick sludge at bottom of ampoule. Patients on self administration must learn to warm the container and shake it thoroughly before injecting). Posterior pituitary snuff may be inhaled 2–3 times daily but is intensely irritant to mucosa causing rhinitis, pharyngitis and even tracheitis and gastritis. 8-lysine vasopressin, a synthetic substitute, may be inhaled from nasal spray 30–60 mg daily.

Thyroid gland: Disorders of thyroid gland

Benign goitre
Enlargement of thyroid gland without oversecretion of thyroxine.

Cause. Continual lack of iodine in drinking water and food reduces thyroxine production, which causes an increase in secretion of thyrotrophin from anterior pituitary gland. Excess thyrotophin causes hyperplasia of thyroid gland.

Types. (1) *Adolescent*. Temporary enlargement in response to greater demand for thyroxine at puberty. (2) *Endemic*. Lack of iodine in certain areas of the world. (Largely combated today by addition of iodine to salt.) (3) *Colloid*. When iodine deficiency corrected large amounts of colloid are made and stored. (4)

Nodular. Pressure of colloid inside vesicles may cause destruction of cuboid cells. Replaced with fibrous tissue which gives nodular feel. (5) *Cystic*. Vesicles may coalesce due to breakdown of intravesicular cells.

Signs and symptoms. Swelling of neck may be only symptom. May press on trachea causing dyspnoea especially when lying flat. Retrosternal goitre may cause dyspnoea, respiratory stridor, dysphagia. Attack can be fatal.

Treatment. Small soft new goitres tend to disappear on administration of iodine. Lugol's iodine 0·5–1 ml daily in divided doses. Old, established goitres will not regress. Iodine should be administered with great caution as the greatly increased amount of tissue will take up large quantities of iodine and convert to thyroxine while the blood levels of thyrotrophin are high. Very small doses 0·1 ml may be given on alternate days. As output of thyrotrophin falls, doses can be increased.

Retrosternal goitre should be excised.

Complications. Pressure on surrounding structures — trachea, oesophagus, recurrent laryngeal nerve. Haemorrhages into vesicles especially in cystic type — characterized by sudden asymmetrical enlargement of gland. Thyrotoxicosis.

Hypothyroidism
Undersecretion of thyroxin.
Types. 1. *Congenital* (*cretinism*).
2. *Adult* (*myxoedema*).

Cretinism
Cause. Insufficiency of thyroxine due to (1) failure of thyroid gland to develop; (2) failure of pituitary gland to secrete thyrotrophic hormone; (3) maternal iodine deficiency during pregnancy; (4) in some cases — failure to convert colloid into thyroxine in spite of higher than normal ability to take up iodine.

Signs and symptoms. Often missed until child is about 6 months old but keen observation may detect them much earlier. Skin — coarse, dry, sallow; hair — scanty and dry; eyes — narrow, slit-like and set wide apart; nose — broad and flat; mouth — wide pendulant lower lip; tongue — large and protruding; neck — short, thickened with pad of myxoedematous tissue across shoulders; back — lordotic; appearance — cross; temperament — sullen, lethargic, disinterested.

THE ENDOCRINE SYSTEM 139

Others — umbilical hernia common. Pot belly. Constipation. Delayed growth, dentition, and closure of fontanelles. Temperature subnormal. Pulse slow.

Diagnosis. Low circulating thyroglobulins, T3, T4.

Treatment. Immediate administration of thyroxine or one of several synthetic thyroid equivalents.

The longer diagnosis and treatment is delayed the less chance there is of reversing mental retardation.

Myxoedema

Reduced secretion of thyroxine starting after general growth and mental development has taken place.

Cause. (*1*) *Primary:* Atrophy of thyroid gland (may be result of auto-immune response). Thyroidectomy. Radio-active iodine therapy. Deep X-ray therapy. Excessive iodine ingestion over long period. (*2*) *Secondary:* Lack of thyrotrophic hormone (usually associated with lack of other anterior pituitary gland hormones. (p. 134).

Signs and symptoms. Typical facies — dull uninteresting expression, puffy eyelids, alopoecia outer third of eyebrows, Creamy pallor of skin. Dry, thickened, rough skin. Subcutaneous tissues indurated with fluid containing much protein (hence name — myxoedema. Myxa, Greek = mucus). Hair dry, straight and sparse. Tongue enlarged. Speech slow and slurred. Voice hoarse. Mental dullness, apathy. Disinclination for mental or physical effort. Capillary fragility and tendency to bruise easily. Menstruation prolonged. Pericardial effusion common. Constipation. Subnormal temperature and slow respirations which may be severe enough to cause coma. Occasionally psychosis (myxoedema madness). Normocytic anaemia.

Diagnosis. Confirmed by low metabolic rate. Low plasma protein-bound iodine. Low uptake of radio-active iodine. ECG changes — flattened or inverted T wave. Elevated serum cholesterol.

Treatment. Administration of thyroxine or synthetic substitute. Dosage, small to start, gradually building up to maximum. In patients with cardiovascular disease or over 40 years dosage built up very slowly. Angina pectoris and congestive cardiac failure can suddenly become much worse if blood levels of thyroxine suddenly raised. Maximum effect of hormone not reached for 7–10 weeks after commencement and effect lasts several weeks after administration stopped.

Complications. Untreated case. Myxoedemic coma with carbon dioxide narcosis due to excessively slow rate of respiration and circulation. (Treated with fast acting hormone; e.g. triiodothyroxine 0·1 mg and artificial respiration).

Intercurrent infections — tuberculosis, myocarditis, nephritis. *With treatment.* Excessive weight loss, tachycardia, myocarditis.

Hyperthyroidism

Oversecretion of thyroxine. Women more than men (10:1).

Causes. Adenoma of thyroid gland. Oversecretion of thyrotrophin. Possibly a thyroid stimulating hormone other than thyrotrophin (source and nature suspected but not proved). Occasionally (rarely) thyroid tissue present in ovary. Occasionally follows iodine therapy in endemic goitre.

Terminology. Graves' disease. Basedow's disease — after doctors first describing syndrome. Toxic goitre where previously benign goitre oversecretes. Thyrotoxicosis — literally, poisoning with thyroxine. Exophthalmic goitre — signs and symptoms accompanied by protrusion of the eyes.

Pathology. Thyroid gland usually enlarged, soft and highly vascular. Following iodine administration gland gets even bigger, becomes firm and less vascular. In long standing untreated cases there are widespread changes in tissues and organs — degeneration of muscles, enlargement of heart, fibrosis of liver, enlargement of thymus tissue, decalcification of bones.

Signs and symptoms. Usually insidious onset. Excitability, fine tremor of hands and tongue, nervousness, insomnia, restlessness, irritability, loss of weight though appetite remains good or excessive, diarrhoea, elevated temperature, sweating, intolerance of heat, dyspnoea, palpitations and tachycardia, occasionally atrial fibrillation and heart failure. Generally nervous symptoms predominate in younger patients and cardiovascular symptoms in older patients. Occasionally sudden onset following psychic trauma — shattering news, severe fright, devastating experience, e.g. rape, plane crash, etc.

Diagnosis. Assay serum T_3 and T_4 levels.

Treatment. Mild cases may recover spontaneously. Aims — to reduce production of thyroxine. Methods: (1) drugs; (2) surgery; (3) irradiation of gland.

Many of symptoms alleviated with beta-adrenergic blocking drugs (see p. 22), which counteract effects of raised adrenalin levels caused by hyperthyroid secretion.

Drugs. For young patients and mild cases drugs alone may be sufficient. Propylthiouracil 100 mg 6 to 8 hourly. Methimazole (Tapazole) 10 mg 6 to 8 hourly. Dosage may have to be greatly increased in nodular goitre. Treatment continued 1½–2 years and then drug gradually withdrawn. Tests of thyroid activity then made and case reviewed.

Side effects of drugs. Suppression of white cell manufacture. Monthly white cell counts performed and if below 1500 mm^3 drug withdrawn. Agranulocytosis occurs in 1 case in 500.

Surgery. Considered for patients under 40 years and those in whom drugs are failing, or producing severe side effects. Also in large goitre or nodular goitre.

Patient treated with drugs until hyperthyroidism controlled (euthyroid state). Iodine added to regime 10–14 days before operations to make gland firm. Nine tenths of gland removed.

Irradiation. Patients over 40 years. (1) *Radioactive iodine.* 120–140 Ci per estimated gram of thyroid tissue to a total of 8–10 Ci. Drug stored in colloid and gradually kills secreting cells. Dose may be repeated in 3–6 months until normal level of thyroxine production achieved.

Complications — radiation thyroiditis. Dangerous in cases with cardiac involvement. Excessive release of thyroxine 5–7 days after administration may cause thyroid crises. (2) *Deep X-ray irradiation.* Now seldom used. Effect is satisfactory but involves lengthy treatment. Poor results in nodular goitre.

General care. Hospitalization not necessary except for initial investigations and pre-operative care or when cardiovascular involvement severe and close observation needed until drug therapy well established.

Patient should continue occupation but warned against over-exertion. Diet rich in protein, carbohydrate, vitamins and calcium. Adequate rest by mild sedation if necessary.

Thyroid crisis (rare)

Sudden severe increase in all signs and symptoms.

Cause. Sudden release of large amount of thyroxine into circulation. Almost always a postoperative complication occurring in patients who have not been prepared adequately with antithyroid drugs. Precipitated by adrenocortical insufficiency. May occur in radio-active iodine therapy.

Signs and symptoms. Intensification of previous symptoms. Extreme irritability, Hyperpyrexia, severe tachycardia with atrial fibrillation and sometimes heart failure, hypotension, vomiting, diarrhoea, delirium, coma.

Treatment. Immediate administration of intravenous glucose 10 per cent hydrocortisone 100–200 mg, reserpine to lower blood pressure, thiamine, oxygen tent, tepid sponging or sterner measures to reduce temperature. Pentothal anaesthetic. Beta blockade prevents thyroid crisis.

Thyroiditis (*rare*)

Inflammation of thyroid tissue.

Types. 1. Specific acute.
        2. Nonspecific acute.
        3. Chronic.

Causes.

Specific acute — spread of infection from upper respiratory tract.

Nonspecific acute — non-infective, cause unknown.

Chronic (Hashimoto's struma) — possibly auto-immune response to patient's own thyroxine.

Signs and symptoms. Specific acute. Redness, heat, swelling and tenderness of neck over thyroid gland. Hyperthyroidism. *Nonspecific acute.* Occurs in middle aged women. Rapid painful swelling of gland. General symptoms of inflammation. Mild hyperthyroidism. Spontaneous recovery. *Chronic.* Mainly middle-aged women. Firm rubbery swelling of gland. Raised serum gamma globulin. Needle biopsy shows replacement of normal secreting tissue with lymphoid and fibrous tissue. Antibodies to thyroglobin found in plasma. Hypothyroidism.

Treatment. Specific acute: Antibiotics and general care of febrile patient. *Non-specific acute.* Nil specific. Inflammation reduced with ACTH gel 80 units daily for one week, or cortisone 50 mg 6 hourly. Codeine or aspirin sufficient analgesic. *Chronic:* Thyroxine.

Neoplasm of thyroid: Benign

Adenoma. Usually occurs in non-toxic goitre; may cause thyrotoxicosis.

Malignant

Malignant adenoma. Metastasizes readily to bone. Often diagnosis made on investigation of metastases. Usually arises in non-toxic goitre.

Adenocarcinoma. Arises in previously unaffected thyroid gland. Grows slowly and invades surrounding structures but does not metastasize to distant parts.

Carcinoma. Rare. Gland previously normal. Rapid or slow growth. Invades surrounding structures and metastasizes to distant parts.

Signs and symptoms. Hard, lumpy enlargement of gland which becomes fixed to surrounding tissues. Pressure symptoms common — dyspnoea. dysphagia, hoarseness. Lymph nodes enlarged in neck.

Treatment. Usually conservative. Occasionally thyroidectomy followed by replacement therapy.

Parathyroid glands: Disorders of parathyroid secretion

Hypoparathyroidism

Reduction of circulating parathormone.

Cause. Usually associated with accidental removal of one or more parathyroid glands during thyroidectomy. Milder cases common starting before puberty and continuing many years. Cause unknown.

Result. Fall in plasma parathormone resulting in low blood calcium, raised blood phosphates.

Signs and symptoms. Tetanic spasm of muscles due to increased sensitivity at neuromuscular junctions in absence of calcium, cramps, twitching and convulsions.

Carpo-pedal spasm (feet and toes extended; elbow, wrists and metacarpo-phalangeal joints flexed with fingers extended).

Lesser degrees may show only fatigue, muscle weakness, palpitation, numbness, tingling in hands and feet. Acute symptoms may be precipitated by infection, menstruation, exhaustion, emotional upsets.

On examination — evidence of increased excitability of muscles. Chvostek's sign — spasm of facial muscles on tapping facial nerve in front of ear. Peroneal sign — dorsiflexion and abduction of foot on tapping head of fibula below knee. Trousseau's sign — carpal spasm after application of tourniquet to upper arm. Skin may be dry and rough; axillary and pubic hair thin and prematurely grey; nails brittle and ridged. Cataract common in later years.

Treatment. Aim: to raise blood calcium levels and maintain at normal. In acute phase — intravenous injection calcium gluconate 10 ml of 10 per cent solution, or calcium chloride 10 ml of 5 per cent solution. Action is short unless parathormone also given, 100–200 units, and then 25–50 units every 6–12 hours. Thereafter, dihydrotachesterol (AT10) 4–6 mg daily until calcium appears in urine and then 1·25 mg 3 to 5 times per week together with calciferol 50 000 to 200 000 units daily and 6 to 8 g calcium daily in the diet.

Hyperparathyroidism

Oversecretion of parathormone.

Cause. Adenoma 90 per cent. Hyperplasia. Carcinoma.

Pathology. Usually one gland only affected. Encapsulated, soft, brown. Embedded in fat.

Signs and symptoms. Muscular weakness, anorexia, nausea, constipation. Polyuria and polydipsia may develop later. Often first clue is renal colic or spontaneous fracture. X-ray shows osteoporosis, cysts, fractures, bony deformities.

Bone marrow depression common with anaemia. leucopenia, thrombocytopenia. Peptic ulcer common. Deafness. Keratitis. Kidney stones.

Diagnosis. High blood calcium. Decreased serum phosphate. Increased urinary calcium and phosphate. Intravenous calcium test — in a normal person a sudden load of calcium causes raised phosphate level in blood and urine. In hyperparathyroidism this does not occur.

Treatment. Force fluids. Restrict calcium intake. Explore surgically to locate and remove affected gland. In general hyperplasia all except one gland removed. Postoperatively a large calcium intake is needed as bones take up calcium very rapidly as soon as parathormone level drops.

Pancreas

Insulin. Passed directly into blood stream where it acts as carrier substance to transport large glucose molecules through small pores of cell membranes. Lack of insulin causes accumulation of glucose in blood. Cells maintain their energy by utilizing di-acetic acid instead. Liver desaturates fats and converts proteins for this purpose. Di-acetic acid produced in excess of needs and constitutes a poisonous substance causing acidosis (ketosis). Proteins not available for cell building so growth and development delayed.

Diseases of pancreas

Diabetes mellitus

Accumulation of glucose in blood characterized by polyuria, polydipsia and reduced resistance to infections.

Causes. (1) Lack of insulin. (2) Development of anti-insulin substances.

Pathology. Early invasion of beta cells with glucose. Fibrosis of pancreas in some cases. Lack of insulin causes greater mobilization of glycogen in liver. This increases blood levels of glucose which may be sufficient for metabolism of cells in mild diabetes. As soon as blood level exceeds 180 mg per cent, glucose lost in urine which offsets the benefits of high blood levels. Tissue need for energy sources causes increased breakdown of fats to diacetic acid. Acidosis (ketosis) results. Increased glucose and diacetic acid in urine prevents reabsorption of water by tubules hence — polyuria and polydipsia with dehydration.

Types of diabetes. (*1*) *Pre-maturity onset:* Patient under 25. Characterized by true insulin deficiency. (*2*) *Maturity onset:* Patient over 25. Characterized by high level of insulin in blood but its action is blocked by anti-insulin factors (not yet identified). (*3*) *Associated with other hormone diseases:* Excess hormones from other glands have anti-insulin effect — growth hormone, thyroxine, adrenaline.

Signs and symptoms. (*1*) *Chronic state:* May be unrecognised for years, then degenerative changes occur and lead to diagnosis — cataract, chronic nephritis, gangrene of toes, arteriosclerosis, cerebro-vascular accidents. (*2*) *Subacute state:* Pruritus, skin infections, moniliasis of vagina, constipation, dizziness associated with dehydration, polyuria, polydipsia. (*3*) *Acute state:* Diabetic coma often precipitated by infection.

Diagnosis. Urine is pale, of high specific gravity (over 1025), contains glucose, acetone (diacetic acid in freshly passed specimen). Fasting blood glucose raised (normal: 3·5–6·0 mmol/l anything over 8·5 mmol/l in fasting subject regarded as evidence of diabetes). *Glucose tolerance test*. Patient prepared by giving 300 g carbohydrate daily for 2–3 days. On day of test, blood taken for fasting glucose level and then 50 g glucose given orally in water. Normally this causes rise of blood glucose to 7·5 mmol/l in first hour but stimulates production of insulin and level falls to below 4·5 mmol/l in second hour. In diabetes level goes on rising to 12 mmol/l or higher, and does not fall in second hour. Test may be performed with intravenous glucose when reference to gastrointestinal absorption is not needed. *Intravenous tolbutamide test*. Fasting blood sugar taken and then intravenous injection of 1 g tolbutamide in 10 ml water. Blood taken for glucose level 20 and 30 minutes later. Normal response — rapid fall of blood sugar due to increased manufacture of insulin. Mature type diabetic response — delayed fall in blood glucose. Prematurity type diabetic response — none.

Treatment. Initial stabilization. Aims. Correction of glucose-insulin imbalance. Maintenance of optimum level of blood sugar, with regard to amount of energy expended, severity and type diabetes.

Patient started on diet and insulin as soon as possible after tests completed. (In severe cases may be necessary to start insulin and diet before tests are completed.) Insulin reserve determined. In prematurity type there is often no reserve and patient needs high doses of insulin daily for life. In maturity type, reserve may be high and patient needs minimal doses of insulin or control may be effected with tablets and diet alone.

Search made for septic foci and corrected if possible — septic teeth, tonsils, gallbladder, sinuses, urinary tract, lungs.

Patient's weight guides initial quantity of food. Prematurity diabetics often greatly underweight; maturity type diabetics often greatly overweight. Ideal weight, for age, height and type of body structure, is taken from tables and initial diet arranged at 25 calories per kilogram of ideal weight. Variations from this will be arranged later taking into account the energy expenditure which will be required for person to carry on his normal activities.

Insulin started at 10 units crystalline insulin daily and subsequent doses determined by level of blood sugar and amount of glucose in urine. At first urine tested carefully 4 times daily — on rising, noon, before evening meal and on retiring. Aim is to keep blood sugar at about 8 mmol/l and to keep urine with a trace of sugar in the specimen immediately preceding insulin injection. Ideally patient has one injection daily. If amount of insulin needed exceeds 40 units per day it is better to have two injections.

Types of insulin

1. Crystalline (soluble, regular). Aqueous solution, clear and colourless. Action starts immediately on injection, reaches peak in about 3 hours, action completed in 5–6 hours.

2. Protamine zinc (PZI). Protamine added in excess to crystalline insulin. Protamine delays absorption and spreads effect over 30 hours. (Must not be mixed with crystalline insulin as the excess of protamine converts some of the crystalline to PZI).

3.Neutral Protamine Hagedorn (NPH). Similar to PZI but amount of protamine added is exactly sufficient to combine with the amount of crystalline. Absorption is delayed and effect continues over 24 hours. Can be mixed with crystalline when both quick and prolonged action are required.

4. Globin insulin. Globin used instead of protamine. Effect similar to NPH insulin.

5. Insulin zinc suspensions. Zinc acetate added. Ultra-lente — similar prolonged action to PZI Semi-lente — action is equivalent to NPH with small amount of crystalline added i.e. immediate action followed by long continued mild action. Lente — mixture of ultra- and semi-lente insulins with action similar to NPH insulin.

It is usual for patients to have a mixture of two of the above, crystalline and a long acting insulin so that effect is continuous. Very large doses of PZI are contra-indicated because of extremely slow rate of absorption. It overlaps the next day's dose.

Insulin reactions. Crystalline insulin causes rapid drop in blood sugar. Meal must be taken within half an hour of injection and must contain sufficient carbohydrate to counterbalance effect of insulin.

Slow acting insulins cause a very gradual fall in blood sugar which is counterbalanced by the normal meals. If insufficient carbohydrate in last meal of day, blood sugar may fall dangerously low during early hours of morning. Patient wakes with headache, nausea, confusion and incoordination. Resembles a mild cerebro-vascular incident and may be mistaken for same, especially in diabetics with hypertension and arteriosclerosis where such an event is not unexpected. Other symptoms — lethargy, sweating, nightmares, palpitation. Patient advised to increase amount of carbohydrate in last meal or to set alarm clock for 2 a.m. and take a snack then. Repeated hypoglycaemic attacks damage cerebral cortex which is to be avoided at all costs. They indicate the need for re-assessment of case with a view to adjusting carbohydrate/insulin balance. Attacks in the late evening or early morning suggest too much long acting insulin. Alternatively there is need for increased carbohydrate in diet especially if attacks are accompanied by weight loss.

Local reactions. May be common at first but tend to disappear. Redness, heat, nodule formation at site of injection. Occasionally there is localized loss of fat and loss of sensation. Generalized sensitivity and anaphylactic shock occurs rarely and usually patient sensitive only to one type of insulin. Changing type, or merely changing brand stops this. Occasionally protamine causes allergy and patient advised to change to globin insulin.

Insulin resistance may occur and requires in excess of 200 units of insulin to maintain control over diabetes. Occurs in conjunction with severe acidosis liver damage and neoplasm. Such resistance usually wanes as time goes on.

Oral hypoglycaemic agents

Useful only in patient with good insulin reserve. If patient can be controlled on 20 units insulin daily he can usually be controlled on tablets instead. Between 20 and 40 units daily he may be controllable with tablets and insulin together. Over 40 units daily and in all prematurity type diabetic tablets should not be used.

Sulphonylureas: tolbutamide, chlorpropamide. Tolbutamide (Orinase, Rastinon, Artosin) 1 to 2 g daily. Chlorpropamide (Diabinese) 250 to 500 mg daily. Abrupt change from insulin to sulphonylurea may be made if patient not receiving more than 20 units insulin daily. Combined sulphonylurea and insulin recommended for patients receiving more than 20 units. Careful observation of reaction must be made with any patient who has complications such as hypertension, liver damage, ketosis, infections, surgical procedures, renal disease and peptic ulcer.

Side effects. Urticaria, vomiting, exacerbation of peptic ulcer, anaemia, leucopenia.

Diet

Aims 1. To supply sufficient food for patient to maintain ideal weight.

2. To supply sufficient calories for energy requirements.

3. To supply sufficient protein for tissue anabolism.

4. To provide as attractive and varied a diet as the restriction on carbohydrates allows.

5. To provide optimum quantities of minerals and vitamins.

Carbohydrates. Approximately 2 g per kg ideal body weight. Increased if patient very active and during childhood. Alternatively amount may be based on 40 per cent of total calories allowed.

Proteins. 1 to 1½ g per kg for adults. 2 to 3 g per kg for children, during pregnancy or when surgery contemplated. At least half of the protein should be first class. In renal impairment this may have to be reduced to ½ g per kg.

Fats. Balance of calories after carbohydrates and proteins have been arranged are met with fats. As little saturated fats, (mostly animal), as possible. Poly-unsaturated fats keep down blood levels of high density cholesterol which is believed to influence development of atherosclerosis.

Meals. Wide range of alternative foods available from modern diabetic diet charts. *Principles*. (1) Three main meals a day with snacks between and before retiring. (2) Bulk of carbohydrates to be contained in meals immediately following injections. (3) Patient must eat all the meal every time. (4) Meal must not be delayed longer than half an hour after injection. (5) Neither meal nor injection to be omitted e.g. because patient does not feel hungry or is not feeling well.

Education of patient for self care.

Ideally patient will manage his own injections and meal entirely. To do so he must have a full understanding of his condition and its control. Details of teaching him is a nursing duty during initial stabilization.

Urine testing. Patient taught method and interpretation of results. He should test his own urine from start of treatment, under supervision at first.

Injection technique. Patient should learn to administer subcutaneous injection. Skin of thighs and abdomen most easily accessible and leaves both hands free. Cleanliness of hands and skin stressed.

Sterilization. Use of single time disposables best. Essential that patient understands risks of carelessness. Simple methods of sterilising using ordinary household equipment taught — saucepan for boiling, covered metal or glass box for storage of syringes and needles.

Insulin. Complete familiarity is necessary especially with the types of insulin ordered. Adequate reserves must be kept in store.

Meals. It may be necessary to weigh portions at first but patients become adept at estimating quantities. Adequate fluid intake also stressed to prevent urinary infections.

Personal hygiene. Mostly a matter of scrupulous cleanliness, avoidance of cuts, scratches, blisters and avoidance of contact with known sources of infection. Feet are particularly important — cleanliness, carefully trimmed nails, well fitting hose and shoes. Corns, fungal infections, deformities of toes should receive regular expert attention.

Diabetic societies. Patient may derive much benefit from belonging to such a group. He will be kept up to date with latest developments, informed of benefits he can receive and meet fellow diabetics for discussion of mutual problems.

Possible complications. Patients should know signs and symptoms of hypoglycaemia. Some doctors allow patient to experience the onset (under close supervision) so that he may recognise the symptoms. Glucose or barley sugar should always be carried so that prompt treatment is available before loss of consciousness.

Need for continued medical care. Patient encouraged to visit doctor regularly. Many complications can be alleviated if they are diagnosed early. Need for prompt medical attention as soon as any infection occurs is stressed.

Complications

Primary. Insulin coma. Diabetic coma.

Secondary. Degenerative changes in small blood vessels leading to retinopathy, neuropathy, nephropathy, gangrene.

Hyperglycaemia

(Diabetic coma, diabetic ketosis). Accumulation of glucose and ketones, (mainly diacetic acid), in blood.

Signs and symptoms. Gradual onset — days or weeks. Increaing weakness and drowsiness. Laboured deep breathing with smell of acetone on breath. Anorexia, nausea, vomiting. Polyuria, polydipsia, dehydration. Possibly fever and abdominal pain.

Due to dehydration — florid dry skin, decreased blood pressure, weak, rapid pulse, reduced eyeball tension, dry brown tongue.

Urine contains sugar and acetone. Blood sugar raised. (Quick reliable method of determining that blood sugar is raised — Ames Dextrostix. One drop of blood allowed to permeate reagent strip for one minute and then washed under a fine jet of water. Colour change shows presence of sugar in blood higher than 7·5 mmol/l.

Treatment. Aims. 1. Immediate administration of insulin to reduce blood sugar.

2. Immediate correction of dehydration and electrolyte imbalance.

3. Immediate treatment of shock consequent on dehydration.

4. Treatment of infection which often precipitates condition.

5. Maintenance of clear airway while unconscious.

6. Restabilization.

Insulin. 100 units given at once. May be given intravenously or, to achieve more prolonged effect, 60 units intravenously and 40 units intramuscularly. If after 1 hour blood sugar is still over 30 mmol/l a further 100 units given intramuscularly. If between 18–30 mmol/l, 50 units given. As soon as blood sugar falls to 12 mmol/l, glucose given to cushion effect of further insulin to ensure that patient does not swing over to hypoglycaemia. It also lessens ketosis more rapidly. Indwelling catheter inserted and hourly specimens of urine tested. Great care needed once blood sugar has fallen to 12 mmol/l. Sugar in urine is reliable guide to glucose/insulin balance at this stage. A rough guide is to give 1 g glucose with each unit of insulin to prevent conversation from hyper-to hypoglycaemia.

Fluids: Water, sodium, chlorides, potassium and phosphorus may all be deficient in hyperglycaemia. Hypotonic saline (0·45 per cent saline) given first. In severe ketosis the acid/base balance can be more quickly restored if sodium bicarbonate is added to saline (15 g per litre). In milder cases sodium lactate solution may be used instead.

The administration of sodium may cause a serious loss of potassium producing weakness, respiratory distress and irregularity of pulse. Corrected by infusing potassium, generally by adding it to glucose solution when blood sugar has reached 12 mmol/l.

Urine output should be carefully measured and charted.

Shock. Low blood pressure and other signs of shock may indicate need for intravenous plasma or whole blood before the above measures will benefit patient's condition. Foot of bed raised. Vasopressor drugs such as noradrenaline (Levophed) 4–16 mg may be added to first flask of intravenous fluid.

As soon as patient able to drink fluids in normal manner without nausea and vomiting, intravenous therapy discontinued.

Patient's airway. During deep coma there is little danger of vomiting but as unconsciousness lightens, danger increases. Many doctors require an intragastric tube to be passed on admission and the stomach aspirated every 15 minutes. As consciousness returns, fluids injected through the tube after each aspiration; each aspiration measured to gauge how much fluid has been absorbed.

Infection. Often precipitates diabetic ketosis. Treated with penicillin 1 mega unit 6 hourly.

When patient has recovered restabilization is needed.

Hypoglycaemia (insulin coma). Fall in blood sugar to below 40 mmol/l.

Cause. Overdosage of insulin. Inadequate carbohydrate after injection. Inadequate glucose reserves to offset long acting insulin. Sudden utilization of glucose by unaccustomed or vigorous exercise.

Signs and symptoms. Sudden onset. After crystalline insulin, onset often about 10·30 a.m. as injections usually given at 8 a.m. With long acting insulins onset usually in late evening or very early morning.

Anxiety, sweating, hunger, headache, irritability, irrational behaviour, fine tremor of hands and tongue, later — twitching or convulsions. Skin pale and moist. Pulse full and bounding. Pupils dilated. Urine free of sugar and acetone. (Empty bladder completely — this specimen may have been in bladder for some hours and may contain sugar. Wait 5 minutes and collect second specimen.)

Treatment. Give glucose at once — orally if possible, or by intragastric tube or intravenously. Recovery is usually sudden, complete and dramatic. Cause of hypoglycaemia should be sought and corrected. Importance of adequate carbohydrate intake to balance insulin must be stressed. Restabilization if attacks are repeated.

Retinopathy

Common complication — as high as 90 per cent in diabetics of 15 years standing. Dilated retinal veins show beading. Capillary haemorrhages may gradually destroy rods and cones. Thickening and fibrosis of vitreous humour with detachment of retina. Cataract common. Made worse by hypertension, atherosclerosis and renal insufficiency.

Nephropathy

Degenerative changes in glomerular capillaries and tubules. Albuminuria may be first indication. Low blood albumin may occur causing oedema. Increases severity of hypertension. Eventual renal or cardiac failure with tendency to thrombosis. (Renal threshold for glucose rises thus making difficulties when urine test for sugar is used as basis for quantities of insulin).

Atherosclerosis

Very common complication occurring about 10 years earlier in diabetics than in non-diabetics. Arteries of heart and legs affected first, causing coronary occlusion and gangrene of toes.

Neuropathy

Numbness, tingling, shooting pains, cramps, muscle tenderness, aching, weakness and paralysis. Absence of sweating, faintness, dizziness. Incontinence of urine and faeces. Severe constipation.

Stricter control of blood sugar levels may reverse changes. Large doses of vitamin B complex and vitamin B_{12}.

Hyperinsulinism

Oversecretion of insulin.

Cause. Adenoma of pancreas. Malignant islet cells. Occurs occasionally in malignancy of other parts.

Signs and symptoms. Hypoglycaemic attacks increasing in severity and frequency. Often associated with long interval between meals or excessive muscular activity. Excessive hunger for carbohydrates. May cause obesity.

Weakness, tremor, nausea, sweating, abdominal pain, faintness, circumoral pallor, palpitation.

Mental reactions — irritability, confusion, aphasia, nystagmus, mania, convulsions.

Repetitions of attacks may cause profound personality changes.

Diagnosis. Fasting blood sugar reduced. Administration of glucose brings blood sugar to normal very rapidly.

Treatment. Subtotal pancreatectomy. Should not be delayed as 20 per cent are due to carcinoma.

Adrenal glands: Diseases of the adrenal glands

Addison's disease (Chronic adrenocortical insufficiency)

Deficient production of cortical hormones.

Cause. Destruction of gland by infections or metastatic invasion, or surgery. Auto-immune adrenalitis. Tuberculosis.

Incidence. Comparatively rare. 1 in 5000 admissions. Any age or sex.

Signs and symptoms. Insidious onset. Increasing tiredness, weakness, anorexia, nausea, vomiting, weight loss. Increased pigmentation of skin which may extend to mucous membranes. More marked in normally pigmented areas, e.g. areola. Quick, deep tanning on exposure to sun. Multiple freckles may appear. Impotence. Amenorrhoea. Depression.

Diagnosis. Low blood corticoids — less than 6 microgram per cent. Urinary 17-hydroxicorticoid low and not increased after injection of ACTH. Serum sodium and chlorides low while serum potassium raised.

Treatment. Hormone replacement therapy. Cortisone 12·5 to 50 mg daily. Taken with food to prevent gastro-intestinal disturbance. Two-thirds of dose taken with breakfast and a third with evening meal to stimulate normal secretion differences. May be too little control over sodium loss with cortisone. Overcome by either high salt diet or addition of corticosteroid with more potent salt retaining ability, e.g. 9-alpha-fluorohydrocortisone (Florinef, Alflorone, Fludrocortisone) 0·1 to 0·3 mg daily orally or monthly injection of oily Percorten or surgical implantation of pellets 8 to 12 monthly. When this additional drug is used patient should have a high potassium diet.

Diet should be high protein, high carbohydrate. Frequent small meals rather than three large ones.

Acute adrenal crisis

Sudden lowering of blood levels of cortical hormones.

Causes. Intensification of chronic state. Haemorrhagic destruction of glands associated with septicaemia. Sudden withdrawal of cortisone therapy.

Signs and symptoms. Shock with low blood pressure, nausea, vomiting, increasing drowsiness, unconsciousness deepening to coma. Dehydration. Occasionally hyperpyrexia.

Treatment. Immediate shock treatment — intravenous saline /5 per cent glucose, vasopressor drugs (Levophed 4–16 mg), oxygen, foot of bed raised, warmth. Hydrocortisone 100 mg intramuscularly or intravenously and 50 mg 6 hourly for 3 more doses. Gradually reduce dosage over next 3 days until maintenance dose reached.

Complications. Overhydration causing oedema and hypertension, cerebral oedema may cause unconsciousness, pulmonary oedema causes dyspnoea, cyanosis, excessive sputum production.

Potassium loss may be excessive and should be countered by oral potassium chloride 3 to 6 g daily.

Occasionally — psychotic reactions.

Cushing's syndrome

Oversecretion of cortisone.

Cause. Adenoma or carcinoma of adrenal gland. Hyperplasia of gland of unknown cause. Occasionally oversecretion of ACTH due to adenoma of pituitary. Rarely — cortisone-like substance produced by carcinoma elsewhere in body.

Signs and symptoms. Typical general appearance — round, fat face with mouth curving down at corners; fine downy growth of hair on face, forehead and upper trunk; increased weight due to peculiarly distributed deposits of fat — upper face, between shoulders and in the omentum; purple striations on skin of abdomen due to breaking down of dermal collagen exposing vascular bed of subcutaneous tissue.

Muscular weakness. Rapid onset of fatigue. Hypertension. Amenorrhoea and slight masculinity in females; atrophy of testicles in males. Patient bruises readily.

Personality changes in two thirds of cases — irritability, confusion, depression, suicidal tendencies.

May be significant oversecretion of aldosterone with sodium retention and consequent oedema and potassium loss. In 25 per cent of cases — diabetes with resistance to insulin. Osteoporosis and spontaneous fracture occasionally.

Diagnosis. Raised urinary 17-hydroxycorticoids. Level of hydrocortisone in blood remains elevated following a 3–4 day course of dexamethasone. X-ray following retroperitoneal or perinephric gas insufflation may reveal tumour.

Treatment. Bilateral adrenalectomy followed by cortisone therapy as in Addison's disease. When condition is definitely due to pituitary tumour — extirpation of pituitary gland.

Metyrapone (Metopirone) blocks production of cortisol. Doses of 250 mg to 1 g. q.i.d. reduce cortisol to 300–400 nmol/L.

Useful drug to prepare patient for later surgery. In inoperable cases cortisol production completely blocked and replacement therapy with prednisolone given according to need.

Hyperaldosteronism

Oversecretion of aldosterone.

Cause. Adenoma of adrenal cortex. Rarely carcinoma.

Signs and symptoms. Two groups — those associated with low blood potassium and those associated with sodium retention.

(1) Muscle weakness, partial paralysis, tetany, polyuria, polydipsia. (2) Hypertension, headache, enlarged heart, retinopathy, congestive cardiac failure, renal failure.

Diagnosis. Low serum potassium. Raised serum sodium. Persistently alkaline urine. Decreased sodium in sweat and saliva.

Treatment. Excision of adenoma if possible. Bilateral andrenalectomy with hormone replacement for life as in Addison's disease (p. 154)

In inoperable cases spironolactone (Aldactone) 200–400 mg daily may correct hypokalaemia and hypertension but side effects — menstrual irregularity, impotence, gynaecomastia — may be intolerable. Amiloride (Midamor) may be used instead.

Prognosis. Without treatment other than potassium replacement patient dies from renal or cardiac failure. With treatment, progress depends on time elapsed since onset of disease and severity of cardiac and renal damage.

Virilism

Oversecretion of one or more sex hormones by adrenal glands.

Cause. (1) Adenoma. (2) Carcinoma (rare). (3) Lack of specific enzymes concerned with manufacture of aldosterone from stage of chemical similar in structure to sex hormones.

Types. *Congenital*. In female babies — hypertrophy of clitoris, thickening of labia majora, atrophy of labia minora, growth of pubic hair while an infant. In male babies — growth of penis and pubic hair while an infant, rapid bony and muscular growth so that child is much bigger and stronger than his contemporaries but growth stops at an early age and by puberty he is shorter than others of his age.

Pre-pubertal onset. In females — enlargement of clitoris, failure of breast development and menstruation, pubic hair has male distribution, acne. In males — early sexual development.

Adult onset. Rarely a 'pure' oversecretion in adults, usually associated with Cushing's syndrome. In females — masculinization, deepening of voice, heavier features, growth of hair on face and chest.

Treatment. Suppression of ACTH with maintenance doses of cortisone or prednisolone or dexamethasone to reduce patient's output of cortical hormones. Markedly altered genitalia in females may require surgical correction. Adult type treated as Cushing's syndrome (p. 155).

Adrenal steroids. (Large number of proprietary names).

Cortisone. Dosage 5 to 400 mg orally or intramuscularly

depending on reasons for administration. Maintenance dose in Addison's disease 12·5 to 50 mg daily.

Hydrocortisone. Water soluble — Solu-Cortef. Dosage 5 to 50 mg. May be injected directly into joints. Intravenous dose up to 250 mg.

Dexamethasone. Dose 5 to 10 mg daily.

Prednisone. Dose 10 to 100 mg daily.

Prednisolone. Dose 10 to 100 mg daily.

Methyl prednisolone. Dose 10 to 20 mg daily.

Triamcinolone. (Similar to Dexamethasone).

Betamethasone. Dose 0·5 to 1 mg daily (orally).

Fluorohydrocortisone. Dose 1 to 2 mg daily. Maintenance 0·1 to 0·2 mg daily.

Deoxycortone. 2 to 5 mg orally; 2 to 10 mg sublingually, 100 to 400 mg implantation.

Choice of preparation depends on effects required. Some have powerful salt retaining properties, others do not. All are relatively safe for short term treatment but all carry possibility of serious side effects for long term therapy (development of Cushing's syndrome from depression of ACTH); hypertension; perforation and bleeding of peptic ulcers; osteoporosis; aggravation of diabetes mellitus; rapid spread of infections; flare up of old tuberculosis; psychological disturbance; obesity; water retention. Sudden withdrawal may cause adrenal crisis.

Regular checks of weight, blood pressure, urine for sugar, ECG, bone density by X-ray, faeces for occult blood — necessary for any patient on prolonged therapy.

Uses other than hormone replacement. Rheumatoid arthritis — reduction of inflammation and pain, increased movement. Acute rheumatic fever — abatement of symptoms especially pain. Bronchial asthma especially status asthmaticus. Nephrosis. Haemolytic anaemia. Ulcerative colitis. Chronic inflammatory condition of eye and skin.

Phaeochromocytoma

Oversecretion of adrenaline and noradrenaline.

Cause. Tumour of adrenal tissue either within adrenal glands of associated with sympathetic chain of ganglia.

Signs and symptoms. Variable. Depends on amounts secreted and whether secretion is continuous or intermittent. Hypertension — sustained or paroxysmal causing headache, dizziness, nausea, vomiting, sweating, slow pulse. Weight loss. Visual disturbance. Severe attack may terminate in pulmonary oedema, ventricular fibrillation, cerebral haemorrhage.

Diagnosis. Hypertension persists on lying flat. Elevated catecholamines in blood and urine. Histamine provokes attack of hypertension. Phentolamine 0·5 mg intravenously causes rapid but temporary fall in blood pressure. X-ray may reveal mass or displaced kidney.

Treatment. Surgical removal of tumour. May require extensive exploration to find all tumour masses. Severe fall in blood pressure may follow surgery and noradrenaline should be on hand. Phenoxybenzamine (Dibenzyline) 10 to 30 mg daily, gradually introduced, blocks action of catecholamines on alpha receptors.

The gonads: Disorders of the ovaries

Ovarian hypofunction
    Reduction of secretion of ovarian hormones.
Causes. 1. Primary disease of ovary (frequently one ovary only is affected and the other increases secretion under influence of a greater secretion of gonadotrophins so that no signs and symptoms occur).

2. Both ovaries may be affected and may fail to develop, e.g. from virus infections — measles, mumps, — from surgery, X-ray irradiation.

3. Insufficient gonadotrophins.

4. Menopause.

Types. (1) Pre-pubertal. (2) Post-pubertal. (3)Menopausal.

Pre-pubertal. Signs and symptoms. Failure to develop secondary sexual characteristics — breasts especially. Failure to menstruate. Sterility. Continuation of growth of long bones due to persistence of epiphyseal discs. Other hormonal disturbances often associated — diabetes, adrenal hypofunction, myxoedema, virilism.

Post-pubertal. Signs and symptoms. Amenorrhoea. Sterility. Partial atrophy of genitalia and breasts. Osteoporosis.

Menopausal. Signs and symptoms. Irregularity of menstruation at 45–55 years — amount, frequency, duration. Eventual amenorrhoea. Gradual regression of breasts, vagina and uterus. Sparsity of pubic and axillary hair. Vasomotor disturbances — hot flushes. Emotional instability, irritability nervousness.

Treatment. Oestrogen replacement therapy (e.g. ethinyl oestradiol 0·1−0·25 mg daily for 3 weeks followed by one week's rest). Brings about sexual maturation but sterility remains. Treatment in menopausal hypofunction — nil unless emotional upset is disturbing, then, mild sedation.

Ovarian hyperfunction

Oversecretion of ovarian hormones.

Causes. Tumours of hypothalamus. Tumours of the ovaries, (May be benign or malignant).

Types. (1) Pre-pubertal. (2) Post-pubertal.

Pre-pubertal. *Signs and symptoms*. When amount of hormone is normal there is premature onset of puberty, rapid skeletal growth which finishes early so that the child is much taller than other girls of similar age but at 15−16 years is smaller than her contemporaries. Early onset of menstruation and ovulation. (Conception is possible).

When amount of hormone greatly in excess of normal there is the same early maturation but inhibition of ovulation occurs and prevents conception.

Post-pubertal. *Signs and symptoms*. Abnormalities of menstruation — frequent (metrorrhagia), excessive (menorrhagia), irregular.

Treatment. Removal of ovarian tumours.

Disorders of the testes

Hypogonadism

Lack of development of testicular tissue concerned with production of testosterone.

Causes. Lack of luteinising hormone, more appropriately called interstitial cell stimulating hormone (ICSH), in males. Undescended testes. Klinefelter's syndrome. Froehlich's syndrome. Destruction of testes by disease, surgery or trauma.

Types. (1) Pre-pubertal. (2) Post-pubertal.

Pre-pubertal. *Signs and symptoms*. Failure to develop male secondary sexual characteristics. Persistance of high voice. Partial or total lack of body and facial hair. Small penis and prostate gland. Continuation of bony growth beyond normal time of closure of epiphyseal discs. Deposition of fat resembling breasts.

Delay in diagnosis common. When both testes are undescended condition is inevitable unless one can be brought into scrotum before age of 12.

Post-pubertal. Signs and symptoms. Secondary sexual characteristics do not regress once they are established. Sexual desire and performance gradually decline and prostate gland atrophies.

Treatment. Administration of one of the long acting synthetic testosterone substitutes. 150 mg intramuscularly every 3–4 weeks gradually increasing to 250–300 mg monthly. Overdosage indicated by acne, hirsutism, retention of sodium with oedema, aggressive personality. When fault is pituitary tumour, gonadotrophins may be used — 500–1000 units 2 or 3 times weekly.

Hypergonadism

Oversecretion of testosterone.

Causes. Testicular tumour — carcinoma or Leydig cells. Excessive secretion of adrenal androgen. Tumour of hypothalamus.

Signs and symptoms. Little or no change in adults. Prepubertal — early sexual development. By 3–4 years child may have adult sexual organs, growth of body and facial hair, deep voice. Bony growth is very rapid but stops at early age.

Treatment. Surgical removal of tumours. X-ray irradiation. Methotrexate reported to have favourable effect on some forms of testicular tumour.

6. Bones and Joints

Disease of bones

Osteoporosis

Decrease in proportion of calcium phosphate in bones.

Causes. (1) Disuse of bones, e.g. in prolonged bedrest. (2) Calcium deficiency in diet. (3) General malnutrition especially protein deficiency coupled with diabetes and hyperthyroidism. (4) Endocrine disorders causing suppression of osteoblast activity e.g. Cushing's syndrome, overactivity of adrenal glands. (5) Bone tumours.

Signs and symptoms. Pain in bones. Gradual deformity. Spontaneous fracture. Muscular weakness. Early onset of fatigue. Renal calculi.

Diagnosis. X-ray shows diminished density of bones.

Treatment. 2–3 g calcium daily. In females, oestrogen may be given post-menopausally, e.g. ethinyl oestradiol 0·1–0·25 mg daily. (In senile osteoporosis, vitamin D is contraindicated as it induces high blood levels of calcium and renal calculi). When bedrest must be prolonged calcium witheld as it will not be incorporated into bones. It remains in blood and is excreted by kidneys where it can cause calculi.

Rickets and osteomalacia

Insufficient calcification of bones.

Causes. (1) Vitamin D deficiency. (2) Calcium deficiency. (3) Inability to absorb sufficient calcium, e.g. in coeliac disease and ulcerative colitis. (4) Excessive excretion of calcium in urine. (5) Excessive loss in milk during lactation without adequate replacement, especially when pregnancies succeed each other rapidly.

Pathology. Proportion of matrix to calcium phosphate excessive.

Signs and symptoms. In adults — anorexia, weight loss, pain in bones, muscular weakness, renal calculi, pyelonephrosis, urinary tract infections. In children — irritability, restlessness at night, beading of ribs at costosternal junctions. In severe cases — bone deformities, e.g. retraction of sternum, softening of cranial bones, box-shaped skull, bowing of legs, pot belly due to laxness of muscles, tetanic spasms.

Diagnosis. Raised plasma alkaline phosphatase. (X-rays may fail to reveal calcium deficit in bones until it is severe).

Treatment. Correct cause. Supply vitamin D and calcium. Calciferol 25 000–100 000 units daily until plasma alkaline phosphatase is normal and then maintenance doses of 5000 units daily. In acidosis loss of calcium in urine is severe. Corrected by administration of sodium citrate, sodium lactate or calcium gluconate which encourage reabsorption of calcium from renal tubules. Calcium salts and vitamin D encourage absorption in intestines.

Paget's disease (Osteitis deformans)

Chronic condition occurring over 50 years of age in which softening of bone is followed by new calcification and hardening. This results in deformities, notably enlargement of cranial (not facial) bones, spinal curvature and bowing of tibiae.

Cause. Unknown. Associated with atherosclerosis.

Pathology. Vasodilation in affected areas. Increased fibrosis. Decalcification and new bone formation goes on simultaneously and repeatedly. Affected bones tend to fracture spontaneously.

Signs and symptoms. Slow onset often without symptoms. Warmth over affected areas. Bone pain — deep, aching and persistent. Headache. Enlarged cranium noticed when hats become too small. Curvature of spine. Diminished height due to bowing of tibiae.

Spontaneous fracture may be first indication. Often patient comes for investigation regarding pain in one knee due to arthritic changes. On examination it is found that Paget's disease affects the other leg and the patient has been unconsciously favouring that side and putting a strain on the other knee.

Diagnosis. Confirmed by X-ray skeletal survey. Bones most commonly affected in this order — cranium, tibiae, pelvis, vertebrae, femora, humeri. Serum alkaline phosphatase raised. Urinary calcium high.

Treatment. *1. While patient able to walk*. High calcium intake, a pint of milk a day. Keep patient as active as possible to stimulate bone development and delay deformity. Anabolic steroids may be given, e.g. testosterone (Deladumone). Cortisone may be used initially if high blood calcium is affecting heart but stopped as soon as possible as it may induce osteoporosis. Vitamin C in high doses may reduce pain. Salicylates give good analgesia. *2. When patient immobile in bed*. Aim is to reduce blood calcium and prevent renal calculi. Dietary calcium, phosphorus and vitamin D reduced. Sodium phytate given with diet. This forms compounds with calcium in intestine and reduces absorption. High fluid intake keeps urine dilute and prevents crystallization of calcium in kidneys. Raised blood calcium may be treated directly with intravenous dextrose, saline and citrate. Calcitonin (thyrocalcitonin) recently used with excellent results in active Paget's disease.

Complications. Spontaneous fracture. Renal calculi. Heart failure due to high cardiac output.

Osteomyelitis

Infection in bone. May be introduced directly — compound fracture, gunshot wounds, surgery — or blood borne especially if bone immature or injured.

Signs and symptoms. Sudden onset of pain with overlying redness, heat, exquisite tenderness. Pyrexia. Rigors. Limitation of movement due to muscle spasm (pseudo paralysis).

Diagnosis. Blood culture may grow *staphylococcus aureus* (75 per cent), group A *beta haemolytic streptococci* (20 per cent) *staph. epidermidis, strep. pyogenes, strep. faecalis, chlostridium, E. coli*. Raised ESR. Leucocytosis. Anaemia. X-ray may be indefinite at first. Later, bone destruction and subperiosteal new bone formation.

Treatment. Immobilize affected part. Antibiotics of suitable sensitivity as soon as cultures grow but initially broad spectrum drugs used methcillin, oxacillin, nafcillin, cephalosporin, polymixin B, carbenecillin, gentomycin. Operative care may become necessary. Aspiration of soft tissue abscesses, decompression of medullary cavity abscess.

Prognosis. With early diagnosis and adequate antibiotic care, full recovery likely especially in the young. If diagnosis delayed chronic osteomyelitis with bone destruction, deformity and joint involvement can occur.

Chronic osteomyelitis.
Signs and symptoms. Intermittently discharging sinus. May be recurrent pain. X-ray shows isolated areas of necrosis (sequestra) and new bone formation (involucra). May be long periods of quiescence.
Treatment. Suitable antibiotics. Drainage of abcesses. Intermittent imobilization when required.

Neoplasm of bone
Types. 1. *Primary.* 60 per cent of cases — sarcoma of osteoblasts. Others — chondrosarcoma of cartilage, fibrosarcoma, lymphosarcoma, liposarcoma.
2. *Metastatic.* Blood borne carcinoma from any other focus, commonly lungs, stomach, prostate.

Both types cause bony destruction and new bone formation (c.f. Paget's disease). The rate at which these progress determines whether bone deposition (osteoblastic tumour) or bone destruction (osteolytic tumour) predominates.
Signs and symptoms. Pain may be very severe. High blood calcium in osteolytic tumour. High urinary calcium. Renal calculi. X-ray of affected bone shows rarefaction or increased density surrounded by normal bone tissue. Spontaneous fracture common. Swelling and deformity in osteoblastic tumour.
Treatment. Curative amputation but diagnosis is rarely made early enough for this. Palliative treatment — irradiation to impede progress of tumour. Encourage exercises to stimulate bone formation. Analgesics.

Achondroplasia
Congenital defect of epiphyseal discs.
Cause. Unknown.
Signs and symptoms. Extreme shortness of long bones especially humeri and femora. Trunk and head normal size. Height usually about 4 feet. Fingers of equal length and spread apart. Feet large and flat. Sacrum tilted forward. Muscular development excessive for size of bones. Great strength and agility.
Treatment. None.

Diseases of joints and tendons

Ankylosing spondylitis (Marie-Strumpell disease)

Condition resembling rheumatoid arthritis in its effects on joints but with significant differences in distribution and aetiology. Almost always the vertebral joints and sacro-iliac joints affected, rarely any others. Men more than woman (4:1). Onset in young age group, 20–30 years.

Cause. Unknown. Definite inheritance factor involved.

Signs and symptoms. Pain on moving lumbar spine or sacro-iliac joints. Increasing stiffness. Diminished lordosis of lumbar spine. Pain disappears when bony ankylosis occurs. Muscle wasting. If costovertebral joints affected — pain on deep inspiration. X-ray shows diminished joint spaces, calcification of spinal ligaments, porosis of vertebral bodies. ESR raised. Condition may spread to other joints, e.g. shoulders and hips.

Treatment. Hot packs over affected areas. Bedrest with traction when spinal nerve roots compressed. Salicylates in largest tolerable doses. Phenylbutazone very effective but used with caution when it is to be continued for weeks (risk of bone marrow suppression). Deep X-ray therapy often markedly effective — daily irradiation for two weeks — but risk of leukaemia increased x 20). Position of patient important to prevent permanent flexion deformity of spine — sleep flat on back with one pillow on a firm unyielding mattress. Small cushion under lumbar spine. Spinal support fitted for daytime use.

Complications. Aortic insufficiency. Spinal deformity.

Osteoarthritis (Degenerative joint disease — DJD)

Chronic degeneration of articular cartilage and hypertrophy of underlying bone.

Causes. Cumulative trauma hence disease of advancing years.

Pathology. Articular cartilage shows progressive changes — opacities, furrowing or grooving, fraying and ulceration. Underlying bone proliferates and may penetrate cartilage as a dense highly polished surface. Outgrowths of new bone occur at joint margins — lipping. Fibrosis of capsule with contraction later and limitation of movement.

Signs and symptoms. Joint pain and stiffness. Pain usually mild and worse after exercise. Stiffness most marked after rest and relieved by exercise. Most commonly affected joints —

knees, hips, shoulders, distal phalangeal joints. No general con-
stitutional signs and symptoms.

Treatment. Acceptance of condition by patient. Explain that
condition is not crippling. Rest affected joints as much as possible but exercise should be taken within limitations of condition.
Apply warmth in form of infra-red rays. Electric blanket at
night. Avoid further trauma to affected joints.

Tendonitis and tenosynovitis

Inflammation of tendons and tendon sheaths (tubes lined with
synovial membrane though which long tendons pass).

Causes. Often in association with rheumatoid arthritis. Often
infective — gonococcal, tubercular.

Signs and symptoms. Pain along course of tendon on contraction of muscle. Stiffness and deformity.

Complications. Fibrosis and adhesion formation leading to
permanent stiffness and deformity.

Treatment. Rest part — splint or plaster of paris. Apply heat
— infra-red. Analgesics — paracetamol. Local injection of hydrocortisone. Excision of tendon sheath for intractable pain and
severe limitation of movement.

Bursitis

Inflammation of one or more bursae with oversecretion of serous fluid.

Cause. Acute or chronic trauma.

Sites. Any of the 140 bursae can be affected. Most commonly
— deep — subacromial subgluteal, calcanean: superficial —
olecranon, prepatella, ischial.

Signs and symptoms. Pain, sudden in onset, swelling, acute
tenderness worse on movement.

Treatment. Immobilize, Mild analgesics. Gentle exercise to
prevent stiffening. Local injection of procaine.

Complication. May become chronic.

Gout

Serum uric acid raised (hyperuricaemia), due to overproduction or underexcretion or both. Uric acid derived from purine
metabolism.

Types. Primary. Inherited metabolic fault. Secondary. Associated with excessive breakdown of purines, e.g. in myelo-

proliferative disease, treated leukaemia, myeloma. In association with chronic renal disease, thiazide diuretic intake, lead poisoning.

Pathology. Inflammatory and degenerative changes in joints due to deposition of sodium urate crystals. Deposition of chalky material in other tissues — tophi: cartilage of ear, tendons, eyelids. Deposition in kidney collecting tubules may lead to pyelonephritis and calculi. Atherosclerosis and hypertension more common in patients with gout.

Signs and symptoms. Acute attack usually initiated by physical stress, e.g. severe exercise, exposure to cold, acute infection. Severe pain usually in one joint and most commonly in metartarsophalangeal joint of great toes. Attacks recurrent with complete freedom from pain between. Untreated, attack lasts about two weeks. Joint red, swollen and exquisitely tender. Accompanied by pyrexia, malaise, tachycardia, leucocytosis, raised ESR, raised serum urates.

Diagnosis. Confirmed by sudden onset of attack, severity of pain, raised blood uric acid, rapid response to colchicine. X-ray shows little change in early attacks. In chronic gout — destructive changes and punched out areas of reduced density adjacent to joints.

Treatment. *1. Acute attack*. Colchicine 0·5–0·6 mg hourly until pain subsides or until onset of gastro-intestinal side effects: nausea, vomiting, diarrhoea. Tolerable dose level found by trial and error, varies between 4–10 mg daily. Phenylbutazone (Butazolidine) 0·4 g initially and 0·1 g 4 times daily for 2–3 days. ACTH gel 100 mg daily until symptoms subside then gradual reduction of dose (sudden withdrawal may precipitate an attack of gout).

Until pain abates patient should rest in bed with affected joint immobilized.

2. Between attacks. Encouragement of excretion of uric acid with uricosuric drugs. Probenecid 1–2 g daily. Sulphinpyrazone (Anturan) 200 mg daily in divided doses building up to 400–800 mg daily until blood uric acid level falls below 6 mg per cent, then reducing dose to maintain this level. (Side effects — reactivation of peptic ulcer, leucopenia, mobilisation of uric acid and increased risk of renal calculi). High fluid intake.

Sodium salicylate may be as effective as probenecid and is very much cheaper and should be tried first.

Allopurinol diverts metabolism of purines. Instead of uric acid as end product large quantity converted to xanthine which is soluble and readily excreted in urine. As blood level of uric acid falls, tophi and other deposits dissolve and are excreted. Patient may suffer acute attack of gout when allopurinol (Zyloprim) therapy started and should continue analgesic therapy with BTZ or indocid or colchicine concurrently for 2–3 weeks.

Avoid foods rich in purines: sweetbreads, liver, kidney, brain, sardines, peas, beans, lentils, spinach, asparagus. Fats should be reduced as they encourage retention of uric acid.

7. Diseases due to Dietary Imbalance

Vitamin A

Vitamin A found only in animal tissues but a precursor, carotene, occurs both in plants and animals. Carotene converted to vitamin D in intestines but ability to do so poor in children. Vitamin A soluble in fats and alcohols. Carotene soluble in water.

Units. 1 international unit = 0·3 g purified vitamin A. Carotene has half the activity of vitamin A therefore 0·6 g = 1 international unit.

Occurrence. Vitamin A found abundantly in liver, especially fish liver and most especially in halibut liver oil (0·6 to 1·5 *grams* per 100 *grams* fresh liver). Compare sheep liver — 3 mg per 100 grams.).

Absorption. Vitamin A readily absorbed from intestine in presence of bile salts. Stored in liver. Liver levels fall rapidly to 50 per cent or less in peptic ulceration, endocarditis, septicaemia, chronic nephritis. In pneumonia, loss in urine may be as high as 300 iu per day. Conversion of carotene takes place readily in healthy adults, but not in hypothyroidism, intestinal and liver diseases, diabetes mellitus and phosphorus poisoning.

Functions. *1. Vision*. Vitamin A present in visual purple (rhodopsin), necessary for initiating an impulse when light strikes retina, particularly necessary for vision in dim light. *(2) Epithelium*. Plays a part in maintenance of all epithelium especially health of cilia, keratinization of skin, and clarity of cornea. *(3) Bones and teeth*. Normal density of bones and teeth depends on vitamin A. *(4) Fetal development*. High proportion of stillbirths and hydrocephalus in animals deficient in vitamin A. *(5) Antagonises peripheral effects of oestrogen*. Abates premenstrual tension.

Deficiency diseases
  Night blindness (Twilight blindness, nyctalopia). Resynthesis

of rohdopsin extremely slow. Normally, development of rod vision, which occurs when light is dim, takes from 5 to 8 minutes and called dark adaptation. In vitamin A deficiency it may take an hour or more.

Dryness of skin. Hard lumpy keratinization occurs especially round hair follicles.

Xerophthalmia and keratomalacia. Cornea thickens, becomes opaque and develops white spots.

Retarded growth. Bones do not develop properly. Density of bone increases. Compact bone is thicker. If this occurs around orifices in base of skull, cranial nerves may be subjected to pressure.

Respiratory infections. Sparsity of ciliated epithelium interferes with one important means of keeping lungs clean, hence there is increased tendency for respiratory diseases to occur readily.

Causes of vitamin A deficiency

(1) Insufficient vitamin A (or carotene) in diet. (2) Poor absorption due to inability to absorb fats as in sprue, coeliac disease, regional ileitis, ulcerative colitis. Habitual use of mineral oil to combat constipation reduces intestinal absorption.

Rare condition in affluent countries. May occur in bottle fed babies if milk not supplemented as liver's store is poor at birth.

Treatment

Administration of vitamin A 5000–25 000 iu daily for 6 weeks.

Hypervitaminosis A

In rare instances symptoms of poisoning from vitamin A occur. Usually due to over-enthusiastic self treatment with halibut liver oil capsules over a long period. Revealed by hepatomegaly, splenomegaly, anaemia, falling hair, drowsiness, vomiting, headache. May be alarming but complete regression occurs on cessation of intake.

Vitamin B complex

Vitamin B1 (Thiamine, Aneurin)

A colourless crystalline compound with a distinctive 'nutty' smell.

Distribution. Widely distributed in grains, nuts, green plants especially growing shoots, yeast (and food items in which yeast has been used for leavening), most protein foods. Some manufactured by intestinal bacteria.

Units. 1 international unit = 0·003 mg.

Needs. Children 1–14 years: 0·7–0·3 mg daily. Adults: 1–1½ mg daily.

Actions. Utilized by enzymes during metabolism of proteins, fats and carbohydrates. Also in formation of acetylcholine at synapses and neuromuscular junctions. Nerves and muscles use large amounts.

Vitamin B2 (Riboflavine, Lactoflavine)

A vivid yellow-orange crystalline substance with a bitter taste.

Distribution. All leafy vegetables, lean meat, fish, liver, yeast, milk. Manufactured in large amounts by intestinal bacteria.

Needs. 1·5 mg daily. 2 to 2·5 mg daily during pregnancy.

Actions. Takes part in many oxidation processes in metabolism. Affects development of fetus. Babies born to mothers deficient in vitamin B2 throughout pregnancy may have skeletal deformities such as grossly receding chin, shortened long bones, coalescent ribs, cleft palate.

Avitaminosis B1

Dietary deficiency of vitamin B1.

Causes. (1) Insufficient in diet. (2) Inadequate absorption.

Signs and symptoms. *Initially*. Anorexia, nausea, vomiting.

Later. Lassitude, poor muscle tone, constipation, nervous depression, irritability, poor memory, poor concentration.

Severe deficiency causes beri-beri with either oedema as initial symptom with enlargement of heart and congestive cardiac failure, or dry form in which nervous symptoms predominate — neuritis, muscular atrophy, extreme weakness.

Blood levels if vitamin B1 fall markedly in heart disease and when mercurial diuretics are administered.

Treatment. Thiamine 3–5 mg daily orally (higher doses are not absorbed). 5–25 mg daily by injection in severe cases until improvement occurs then 5 mg orally daily.

Dietary habits should be investigated and faults corrected.

Ariboflavinosis

Deficiency of vitamin B2.

Signs and symptoms. Fissures at corners of mouth with honey coloured exudate. Flattening of papillae of tongue. Photophobia. Dimness of vision. Vascularization of cornea. Cataract. Dermatitis. Pruritus.

Treatment. Increase intake of foods rich in vitamin B2: milk (1 pint per day provides average needs), lean meat, green vegetables.

Prevention. Dietary intake during pregnancy should be increased to 2–2·5 mg especially during last 6 months.

Vitamin B6 (pyridoxine)

Occurrence. Cereal germ, liver, yeast, potatoes, occurs widely but in small quantities in most animal and vegetable tissues. Synthesized in large intestines by intestinal bacteria.

Requirements. About 1 mg daily.

Uses. Protein metabolism — co-enzyme in tissue breakdown and reconstitution. Fats — helps conversion of protein to fat. Involved in maintenance of nerves.

Avitaminosis

Indefinite signs and symptoms. Similar to vitamin B2 deficiency. May arise during treatment of tuberculosis with INAH due to formation of unabsorbable compound.

Nicotinic acid(Niacin)

White crystallin powder with an acid taste.

Occurrence. Yeast, whole grains, liver, small quantities in all tissues except fats. Manufactured in large intestine.

Requirements. About 20 mg daily.

Uses. Concerned in protein and carbohydrate metabolism and cellular uptake of oxygen.

Pellagra

A multiple deficiency disease with insufficient intake of vitamin B complex generally and nicotinic acid in particular.

This is combined with an imbalance in the types of protein eaten. Deficiency of tryptophan (an essential amino acid) contributes, as this substance is used in formation of nicotinic acid in large intestine. Other factors influencing incidence — overexposure to sunlight, alcoholism.

Incidence. Occurs most commonly in people living exclusively on maize.

Signs and symptoms. Excessive pigmentation of skin exposed to sunlight, excessive dryness and cracking of skin, poor healing power, blistering. Chronic inflammation of mucosa of digestive tract with ulceration, pain and severe diarrhoea. Increasingly poor absorption of all digested products with rapid and extreme weight loss and dehydration. Nervous symptoms may be severe but do not always occur — delirium, hallucinations, confusion, extreme irritability.

Treatment. Oral nicotinic acid 150 mg daily in divided doses. High protein diet. Intravenous nicotinamide 100 mg daily. General nursing care is important until symptoms subside. Skin care of utmost importance.

Vitamin C (ascorbic acid)

Occurs naturally in many plants as ascorbic acid. Crystallizes to a white powder with a markedly acid flavour.

Units. 1 international unit = 0·05 mg crystalline ascorbic acid.

Distribution. Widely distributed especially in green plants and citrus fruits.

Needs. Most animals can synthesize their own vitamin C. Primates and guinea pigs cannot. Necessary daily intake 10–100 mg. Optimum probably 75 mg. Excreted in urine, faeces and sweat. Absorption takes place readily in intestine but storage is limited to about 5 g — enough for 2–3 months. Intake over 100 mg daily rapidly excreted in urine.

Scurvy

Disease due to shortage of vitamin C.

Causes. Lack of fresh food especially green vegetables.

Occurrence. Rare. (1) Babies — delayed weaning. (2) Elderly people living alone.

Signs and symptoms. *Early*. Keratosis of hair follicles. Scaly patches on skin. Muscular weakness and rapid onset of fatigue. Pains in back and limbs. Perifollicular haemorrhages. Bleeding gums. *Late*. Loose teeth. Oedema of knees. Flare-up of old tubercular lesions. Breakdown of old scars. Diminished capacity for wound healing. Severe haemorrhages — submucosal, haematuria, haematemesis, anaemia. Heart failure.

Treatment. Administer vitamin C 500 mg daily for 3 days and then 100 mg daily. Investigate and correct reasons for low intake. Patient may need bedrest for week or two with physiotherapy to regain muscle tone. High protein diet.

Vitamin D

Sources. Several closely related compounds identified. In higher animals vitamin D3 is formed from 7-dehydrocholesterol. Other forms, D2 (calciferol) D4, D5, D6, occur in other life forms but can be utilized by human tissues.

Units. Vitamin D3, 1 international unit — 0·025 g. Vitamin D2 1 iu — 1 mg.

Occurrence. Fish liver oils extremely rich in vitamin D, tunny, halibut and cod especially. Sun's action on ergosterol in skin makes vitamin D3.

Absorption. From intestine in presence of bile. 70 per cent of ingested vitamin D excreted in faeces.

Action. Regulates calcium and phosphorus metabolism.

Deficiency diseases
  Rickets and osteomalacia (p. 162).

Vitamin E

Occurs in several forms — tocopherols. Fat soluble. Widespread in many foodstuffs — green leafy vegetables, grains, nuts, animal fats. Not destroyed by cooking. Uses in human body uncertain. Has been used with variable benefit in muscular atrophy, atherosclerosis, angina pectoris, anaemia, menopausal disturbance.

Vitamin K

Occurs naturally in all green plants. Many synthetic substitutes available. Enough for body's needs formed by symbiotic bacteria in large intestine. Bile essential for its absorption.

Action. Used by liver for formation of prothrombin on which blood clotting depends.

Deficiency
  Causes of deficiency. (1) Lack of bile in intestine, e.g. in obstructive jaundice. (2) Lack of synthesis by symbiotes, e.g. fol-

lowing course of intestinal antiseptics which kill off useful as well as harmful organisms. (3) Poor absorption due to intestinal hurry, e.g. in ulcerative colitis.

Signs and symptoms. Low prothrombin level in blood. Tendency to bleed. Positive Hess test.

Treatment. Intramuscular or intravenous injection of vitamin K5–25 mg. Prothrombin level tested after 12 hours. Injection repeated if prothrombin still below normal.

Other uses of vitamin K

Antidote when dicoumarol and phenindione derivatives have been used as anticoagulants. Pre-operatively in obstructive jaundice. 1 mg given to premature infants whose blood clotting mechanism is sometimes deficient. Given in prolonged antibiotic therapy to counteract low production in intestines.

Sprue

A disease in which malabsorption of all foods occurs resulting in multiple deficiency signs.

Cause. Unknown. Possibly virus but not proved. May arise secondarily to many diseases altering structure of intestinal mucosa, e.g. tubercular enteritis, regional ileitis, lymphoma, diverticular of small intestine.

Signs and symptoms. Slow insidious onset. Intermittent diarrhoea. Stools large, soft, frothy, foul smelling, and accompanied by much flatus. Pain, nausea and vomiting. Tiredness and early onset of fatigue. Weight loss may be severe. Cramping of muscles common.

As malabsorption continues, vitamin deficiency signs develop — glossitis, angular stomatitis, anaemia, ascites.

Diagnosis. May be difficult. Undigested fat in stools. Blood levels of all feed elements reduced. Barium meal X-ray may show 'scattering' and 'puddling' of barium in small intestine instead of normal, even, feathery distribution.

Treatment. Rest in bed in quiet, congenial atmosphere free from business worries. Folic acid 5 mg twice daily, orally, until symptoms abate, then 5 mg daily. Diet — high protein with mixed vitamins and iron. Remove patient from a tropical climate if possible. Antibiotics and sulphonamides may improve condition dramatically especially in sprue secondary to some other condition.

Kwashiorkor

Protein deficiency disease of young children.

Cause. Weaning onto a diet poor in essential amino acids. Intestinal parasites worsen condition.

Signs and symptoms. Generalized oedema which usually hides underlying emaciation. Enlarged liver. Child weak and miserable. In dark skinned races skin has reddish tinge and hair is 'rusty'.

Treatment. Cured in early cases if diet improved to contain essential amino acids. Skimmed milk and reconstituted milk powder achieves this readily. Education of mothers does much to prevent condition.

Complications. Heart failure. Kidney failure. Increased susceptibility to infections. Cirrhosis of liver common in later years. Atrophy of pancreas.

8. The Nervous System

Disease of the nervous system: Cerebro-vascular disease

Interruption of flow of blood through vessels of brain.
Causes. Haemorrhage. Thrombosis. Embolism.
Results. Interruption of arterial supply to any part of brain causes anoxia in parts thus deprived. Irreversible changes take place in 3–4 minutes. In haemorrhage there is also destruction of nerve pathways by encroaching blood.
Contributory factors. Atherosclerosis. Atheroma. Hypertension especially sudden hypertension superimposed on weakened vessels. Hypotension predisposes to stasis and thrombosis. Aneurysm. Neoplasm. Septicaemia.

Cerebral haemorrhage

Almost always preceded by hypertension.
Signs and symptoms. Patient usually over 40 years. Sudden onset with symptoms intensifying over 1–6 hours. Headache common. Onset during sleep is rare. Increasing muscular weakness down one side of body. Loss of sensation to pinprick over same area. Slurred speech, confusion. Unconsciousness. Respirations deep and irregular. Pupils dilated and not reacting. Incontinence of bowels and bladder. Pulse slow and full. Face cyanosed and congested.
Diagnosis. Confirmed by lumbar puncture which shows blood CSF. Raised white cell count 15–20 thousand per mm^3. Raised ESR.
Prognosis. Death occurs in 70–75 per cent cases within one month. In survivors some recovery of movement, sensation and speech can be expected as blood clot absorbs.
Treatment. General care of unconscious patient — maintenance of airway, pharyngeal suction, tracheostomy if suction ineffective. Frequent turning to prevent pulmonary complications. Avoidance of oral feeding until swallowing reflex returns.

Careful attention to pressure areas. Prevention of deformities especially foot drop, rotation of femur and flexion deformity of hand. Full range of passive moments to all limbs. On recovery of consciousness — active movements of all unparalysed limbs. Encourage movement of paralysed limbs. Full re-education programme from physiotherapist, occupational therapist and speech therapist.

Prevention. Every effort should be made to keep blood pressure down to normal level with antihypertensive drugs, avoidance of excessive exercise and heightened emotional tone. Avoidance of large meals, foods which are hard to digest, alcohol, tobacco.

Cerebral thrombosis

Almost always preceded by atheroma. Other predisposing factors — aneurysm, infection of ear, sinuses, face, severe toxaemia and septicaemia, low blood pressure.

Pathology. Thrombus may occlude one major artery or may consist of numerous small thrombi. Common sites are where vessels branch. Severity depends on presence of collateral supply and speed with which thrombosis occurs. If it develops slowly there is time for collateral supply to develop. Affected parts become soft.

Prodromal signs. In 80 per cent of cases patient experiences transient disability which depends on affected area, e.g. temporary hemiplegia, paresis in various parts, double vision, blindness, confusion, numbness, headache. Attacks may recur frequently. Stroke may follow one such attack or it may not occur for weeks. Occasionally prodromal signs are not followed by a stroke.

Onset of stroke. 60 per cent occur during sleep or shortly after rising. Patient may awake with complete hemiplegia or this may develop slowly over several days.

Signs and symptoms. Depends on area of brain affected.

Middle cerebral artery. Hemiplegia, loss of skin sensation, loss of speech, loss of appreciation of written and spoken words, visual disturbance.

Anterior cerebral artery. Foot and leg paralysis, paresis of arm, urinary incontinence, loss of memory, mental impairment.

Posterior cerebral artery. Hemianopia, blindness, lack of

co-ordination between vision and movement, inability to identify objects.

Pontine arteries. Inco-ordination of muscular movement, falling to side of lesion, paralysis of eye muscles, paralysis of face, arm and leg on opposite side to that of lesion, dizziness, nausea, vomiting.

Vertebral arteries. Paralysis and atrophy of one half of tongue, paralysis of opposite arm and leg, loss of skin sensation in similar area.

Basilar artery. Paralysis of all extremities, blindness, muscle inco-ordination, drowsiness, apathy, impaired memory.

Cerebral oedema may follow embolism and cause increasing coma, rising blood pressure, slowing pulse, dilated and fixed pupils. Respiratory irregularity and raised CSF pressure.

Treatment. As for cerebral haemorrhage.

Paralysis agitans (Parkinson's disease)

Disease of corpus striatum or subthalamic region occurring in persons of 50 years and over, causing disturbance of voluntary muscle tone, involuntary tremor and characteristic facial appearance and posture. Intellect not disturbed.

Cause. Unknown. Some cases occur after encephalitis. Parkinsonian movements may occur in some patients receiving antihypertensive drugs.

Signs and symptoms. Insidious onset with involuntary tremor in one part gradually progressing to tremor of hands, legs, head and tongue. Features become rigid and expressionless. Posture stooped with shoulders rounded. Gait consists of short steps accelerating to a trot (festinating gait). Muscles rigid. Hands held characteristically in front of body with elbows held close to sides and thumbs and fingers forming a 'pill-rolling' action.

Severity of symptoms made worse by emotional stress — anxiety, tension, unhappiness.

Treatment. Psychological support, encouragement, sympathy, understanding. Intellect not impaired but patient's difficulty in communicating satisfactorily leads to severe depression and withdrawal. Antispasmodic drugs may give some relief. Atropine was long used but newer synthetic drugs are more effective — benzhexol (Artane), procyclidine (Parsidol). Some of the antihistamines also are beneficial — diphenhydramine (Benadryl). Combinations of these and other drugs may be used. Dosage to attain maximum benefit must be just short of toxic levels and established by trial.

Excellent response to levodopa (Larodopa) in some cases. Up to 8 g daily given orally.

Amantadine hydrochloride (Symmetril), 200 mg daily also effective.

Physiotherapy, education in relaxation, radiant heat and massage to tense, painful muscles may help patient towards effective rest. Recently, surgical intervention has given remarkable results in selected cases. Certain areas in globus pallidus or thalamus destroyed.

Prognosis. Without surgery, up to 10 years of gradually worsening muscular spasm and tremor until patient bedridden and helpless. Intercurrent infection common.

Chorea (Rheumatic chorea. Sydenham's chorea)

Auto-immune disease affecting cerebral hemispheres.

Cause. Reaction to antibodies that have been produced to combat streptococcal infection.

Signs and symptoms. Occurs almost exclusively in young persons 5–15 years. Girls more commonly than boys (3:1). Always a history of streptococcal infection 2–3 weeks before. Insidious onset with restlessness, fretfulness, insomnia, increasing muscular clumsiness. Later, jerky involuntary movements. Extent and intensity vary from slight twitching of a limb to convulsive movements of whole body. Facial grimacing common. Muscular weakness variable — some patients can carry on almost normal activities, others can only lie in bed. Disturbance of mentality varies. Most are highly excitable, irritable and emotionally disturbed. Occasional mental derangement. Respirations jerky and irregular. Second and third attacks may occur. Risk of rheumatic heart disease increases with each attack.

Treatment. Rest in bed in a quiet environment free from anxiety and excitement. Dietary intake must be maintained and in severe cases feeding by gavage may be necessary. Violent movements may cause injury so cot sides should be padded and in very severe cases patient nursed on mattress on floor.

Aspirin 0·5–1·5 g daily in divided doses. Phenobarbitone 30 mg 3 times daily to promote rest. Convalescence prolonged and diet should contain high protein, vitamins and iron. Prevention of further streptococcal infections attempted with oral penicillin for some years.

Huntington's chorea

Brain disorder characterized by uncontrollable muscular jerking, facial grimaces and progressive dementia.

Cause. Mendelian inheritance of a factor which does not manifest itself until after 40 years of age. Occasional sporadic cases with no family history.

Signs and symptoms. Gradual onset of muscular twitching, irregular respirations, faulty articulation until speech is unintelligible, bizarre grimaces, peculiar dance-like gait. Dementia progressive with maniacal outbursts. Suicide common.

Treatment. Nil.

Epilepsy

Episodic disturbance of consciousness during which generalised convulsions may occur.

Cause. Unknown. Encephalographic studies reveal direct relationship between changes in electrical potential of brain and occurrence of fit. Heredity plays a part. Occasionally occurs after head injury and brain diseases.

Types

1. *Grand mal* (*major epilepsy*). True epilepsy with loss of consciousness and convulsive fits.

2. *Petit mal* (*minor epilepsy*). Minor loss of awareness without loss of consciousness and without convulsions. More common in childhood but may develop into grand mal with maturity.

3. *Jacksonian epilepsy* (*focal, cortical or partial epilepsy*). Consciousness not lost. Convulsions confined to one group of muscles, one limb or one side of body.

Signs and symptoms. *Grand mal*. Sudden loss of consciousness with convulsions and incontinence. Stages of fit: (*a*) *Aura*. Peculiar feeling or sensation preceding fit. May last seconds or hours. Not always present. Gripping sensation in abdomen, strange noise, flashing lights, numbness, disagreeable odour. Varies in character from person to person. Usually same sensation each time for a particular person. (b) *Tonic stage*. Sudden loss of consciousness. Muscles rigid. Patient falls to ground. Cessation of breathing. Skin becomes cyanosed. Teeth clenched. Eyes turned upwards. May last up to 30 seconds. (c) *Clonic stage*. Convulsive movements of all muscles. Tongue often damaged. Incontinence. Respirations convulsive. Much frothing. Sweating. Ends with deep coma and complete relaxation. (d) *Disorientation*. Recovery of consciousness. Patient disorientated and confused. May commit acts without memory of same afterwards. Will sleep deeply if allowed. *Petit mal*. Momentary loss of awareness. May continue routine acts — walking etc. Eyes may turn upwards and rapid blinking or tremor of eyelids. Expression rigid. Patient recovers and continues as if nothing has occurred. Not incontinent. *Jacksonian epilepsy*. Sudden uncontrollable convulsive jerking of limited extent. No loss of consciousness.

Treatment of major attack. Protect patient from self injury. Remove from danger. Restrain only enough to prevent injury. Place something crossways in mouth to prevent biting of tongue. Loosen tight clothing especially tie. Allow to sleep afterwards if possible.

Accurate diagnosis of lesion of brain helped by careful observation of nature of fit — type of aura, where convulsive movements start and their duration and intensity, presence of residual paralysis.

Treatment between attacks. Intensive investigation to discover causes which might be amenable to treatment — tumour, syphilitic lesion, infective focus, emboli, scar tissue in cortex. Surgical removal may cure or reduce incidence of attacks.

Psychological support essential as many epileptics develop feelings of rejection, inferiority, persecution, self-consciousness and depression.

Drugs available which reduce number of incidents or prevent them altogether — diphenylhydantoin (Dilantin, Mesantoin) 0·2–0·6 g, primidone (Mysoline) 1–3 g, oxazolidinedione (Tridione, Paradione) 0·6–3 g, phensuximide (Milontin) 1–3 g. Sodium valproate (Epilim) 0·5–2 g daily. Phenobarbitone and bromides may still be used for mild cases. It is important that drugs be taken regularly to maintain constant blood level even though there has been no fit for years.

Status Epilepticus

Recurrent convulsions with so little time between that patient does not recover consciousness.

Cause. Unknown.

Signs and symptoms. Typical attacks follow one after the other rapidly and so exhaust patient that death may ensue.

Treatment. Various combinations of barbiturates and anti-epileptic drugs are tried. Usually given intravenously for quick action. Ether anaesthetic may stop attacks temporarily.

Complications. Hyperpyrexia. Circulatory collapse. Nephrosis.

Brain abscess

Localized suppuration within brain.

Cause. Any micro-organism. Commonly blood borne pneumococci or staphylococci. Occasionally contiguous spread from middle ear, mastoid, sinus. May follow fractured skull or other cranial injury.

Signs and symptoms. General — often those of septicaemia — remittent temperature, severe prostration. Local — cerebral compression, nausea, headache, vomiting, slowing pulse rate, rising blood pressure. Focal signs depend on site of abscess.

Treatment. Incision and drainage followed by irrigation with antibiotic solutions. Systemic antibiotics. Treatment of source of organisms.

Multiple sclerosis (disseminated sclerosis)

Multiple lesions in white matter of brain and cord which interfere with function of neurones.

Cause. Unknown. More common in temperate climates and in white races. No sex differentiation.

Signs and symptoms. Depends on sites of lesions. Sometimes insidious onset. Occasionally abrupt. Various paralyses. Remissions common. Abrupt onset more common in younger age group 20–30 years and more likely to affect brain. Insidious onset more common in older age group and more likely to affect spinal cord.

Temporary difficulty in walking or use of arms. Temporary blindness in one or both eyes. Progressive weakness and clumsiness of one or both limbs. Interference with nerves controlling muscles of speech resulting in hesitant, discontinuous or staccato speech. Episodes become longer and more severe, remissions shorter and less complete. Eventually, double incontinence and complete dependence. Muscle spasms cause severe pain. Intercurrent infections common. Intellect usually unimpaired. Euphoria common but occasionally severe depression.

Diagnosis. Chiefly concerned with differentiation from other conditions which may be amenable to treatment — cerebral tumour, spyhilis, encephalitis, subacute combined degeneration of cord.

Treatment. Supportive. Physiotherapy to keep patient mobile and fully employed for as long as possible. Patient rarely informed of diagnosis in early stages as remissions may be long and complete. Eventually, intensive care of skin, bowels and bladder of a bedridden patient.

Syringomyelia

Tubular cavitation of cervical spinal cord which may extend into brain stem and dorsal spine.

Cause. Unknown. Possibly a congenital defect as condition often accompanied by other defects.

Signs and symptoms. Spinal curvature may precede others by many years. Curvature due to enlargement of spinal cord pressing against and weakening of pedicles of neural arch. Onset about 30–40 years. Weakness and wasting of arm muscles. Limitation of movement. Loss of sensation for pain and temperature. Sense of touch not impaired. As cavitation extends vital centres may be involved and cause early respiratory failure and death. Eventually patient totally incapacitated. Intercurrent infections common, especially respiratory and urinary tract infections. Loss of appreciation of pain and heat may result in extensive ulceration especially from burns to hands.

Treatment. Decompression of distended cavity in cord may give temporary relief. No treatment to halt progress of disease.

Careful general nursing required to prevent infection and deformities.

Meniere's syndrome (paroxysmal labyrinthine vertigo)

Disturbance of the eighth cranial nerve.

Cause. Unknown.

Signs and symptoms. Sudden, recurrent episodes of vertigo, nausea, vomiting, nystagmus, tinnitus and progressive deafness. Onset often in fifth decade.

Treatment. Rest in bed during acute attack. Patient finds a particular position in which to lie to prevent nausea. Any movement may initiate attack. Dimenhydrinate (Dramamine) 25–50 mg 3 times daily. Low salt diet. Usually vertigo ceases when deafness complete. Occasionally vertigo continuous and severe unless patient lies still. Severest forms may be treated by division of eighth cranial nerve.

Motion sickness (travel sickness)

Temporary disturbance of balance mechanism.

Cause. Unaccustomed movement of the body which is prolonged for more than half an hour or is intermittent. (Large psychological factor as condition can be induced in susceptible persons by merely observing conditions under which symptoms may arise, e.g. films of ships at sea).

Signs and symptoms. Anorexia, nausea, vomiting, vertigo.

Treatment. Almost impossible to stop once it starts and the motion continues. Will eventually stop automatically. Prevention often effective with antihistamines, mild sedatives or parasympathetic depressants. In severe cases, rest in bed under sedation. Dehydration can be severe, hence intravenous fluid replacement may be needed.

Trigeminal neuralgia

Sudden attacks of severe pain in face, usually of short duration but may be frequently repeated.

Cause. Unknown. Attack often stimulated by mild irritation of a 'trigger' zone — pressure, chilling, sudden movement.

Signs and symptoms. Paroxysms of extreme pain along track of one or more branches of trigeminal nerve (fifth cranial nerve). May be a series of stabbing pains or a sudden burning sensation. May persist for hours and stop as suddenly as it started.

Treatment. Inhalation of trichlorethylene (Trilene) 15–20 drops. Best given before mealtimes so that nutritional state can be maintained. Massive doses of vitamin B_{12}, 1 mg daily for 10 days may bring relief. In prolonged cases, injection of alcohol into ganglion

Facial paralysis (Bell's palsy)

Paralysis of facial muscles on one side.

Cause. Unknown. Often precipitated by chilling, 'draughts' and occasionally trauma.

Signs and symptoms. Sudden onset of complete paralysis of one side of face.

Treatment. Support paralysed muscle with wire from corner of mouth to ear to prevent hyperextension of muscle fibres. Massage and electrical stimulation. Recovery usual within 2–8 weeks but occasionally much longer. Very rarely permanent (except from traumatic interruption). Eye may need protection — castor oil drops at night, lid carefully closed and covered with pad. Oral hygiene important.

Polyneuritis (peripheral neuritis)

Widespread disturbance of sensory and motor nerves with non-inflammatory degeneration.

Causes. 1. Toxic agents — arsenic, benzine, phosphorus, alcohol.

2. Infections — syphilis, diphtheria, viruses.

3. Metabolic — diabetes, gout, rheumatism.

4. Nutritional deficiencies — thiamine, cyanocobalamine.

Signs and symptoms. Various anaesthesias, paresis and paralyses.

Treatment. Find and remove cause. Correct if possible — supply deficient vitamins, BAL in arsenical poisoning High calorie diet with additional B vitamins. Rest in bed and immobilise affected parts. Passive movements and massage until pain subsides then active movements encouraged.

Herpes zoster (*shingles*)

Acute infectious disease of posterior nerve root ganglia and peripheral nerve trunks. Usually unilateral.

Cause. Virus of varicella (chicken pox).

Signs and symptoms. Incubation period 7–14 days. Depends on nerve trunk affected — commonly intercostal, arm, leg or ophthalmic nerves. Neuralgia, pruritis, burning sensation along track of nerve. Rash along same tract progressing through stages — macule, papule, vesicle, scab. Occasionally generalized rash as in chicken pox. Occasionally severe motor disturbance with paralysis. Danger of ulceration of cornea and blindness when ophthalmic nerve affected.

General signs and symptoms — often fever, headache, back rigidity, enlarged lymph nodes.

Treatment. Analgesics to control pain. Sedatives to allay tension. Cortisone may be used especially in ophthalmic cases. Rest in bed during acute phase. Local applications to rash — calamine lotion, sodium bicarbonate paste, collodion paint. Antibiotics have no effect except to prevent secondary infection.

Complications. Most commonly seen in elderly patients with atherosclerosis-postherpetic neuralgia, persistent paresis, secondary infection.

Myasthenia gravis

Marked weakness of muscles and rapid onset of fatigue.

Cause. Excessive activity of cholinesterase at neuromuscular junctions. In 20 per cent of cases tumour of thymus gland discovered.

Signs and symptoms. Rapid fatigue of affected muscles. Commonly face, lips, tongue, but any muscle or group of muscles may be affected including diaphragm. Onset may be seen in eyelids and face only, giving the features a set immobile appearance with eyes half closed and head thrown back in order to rotate eyes downwards in order to see. Choking may occur if swallowing muscles affected. Speech becomes difficult to understand when tongue affected.

With rest, partial recovery of muscles takes place but onset recurs much more quickly as soon as muscles are used again.

Respiratory insufficiency may occur abruptly and need emergency treatment.

Treatment. Anti-cholinesterase drugs. For routine care Neostigmine 15–180 mg orally 4 hourly. (Optimum dose established by trial). Pyridostigmine (Mestinon) 0·6–1·5 mg daily in divided doses. Timing of doses important to avoid episodes of weakness when blood levels fall. Ambenonium chloride (Mytolase) 5–25 mg 4-hourly. Galanthamine and lycoramine under trial.

In acute respiratory attacks — Neostigmine 1 mg intravenously repeated until patient comfortable. Unwanted side effects such as intestinal cramps may be prevented with atropine.

Prognosis. Disease characterized by periods of complete remission followed by more severe attacks. Occasionally there is spontaneous cure but most cases progress and need ever increasing doses of Neostigmine. Some cases are not affected by even massive doses of Neostigmine and spend a miserable life in and out of respirators needing oxygen and tracheostomy. Respiratory infections common.

Myasthenia gravis in the newborn. Children born to mothers with the condition may have a severe attack at birth. Treated with Neostigmine and child recovers completely.

Care of the unconscious patient

Choice of situation. Ideally a single room. Patient should not be left unattended, hence bed should be in a position where constant observation is easy. Air conditioning and heating are an advantage.

Equipment. Emergencies may arise suddenly and the following should be immediately available — oxygen, respiratory suction, tracheostomy set, endotracheal tubes. Other routine equipment — torch, sphygomanometer, mouth gag, tongue depressor, tongue forceps laryngoscope.

Bed. Should be firm, flat, with padded cot sides, without a head piece, adjustable and higher than routine hospital beds. Bedclothes should be minimal and wool blankets forbidden.

Position of patient. Horizontal if condition permits, preferably on side to allow pooling of secretions in cheek. Frequent turning to prevent pressure sores and hypostatic pneumonia.

Airway. Lateral position ensures tongue cannot fall back and prevents inhalation of vomit, blood or saliva. Where dorsal position cannot be avoided, chin should be held forward, no pillow under head. Suction should be carried out immediately before and immediately after changes of position.

Record kept of respiratory rate, depth and character. Difficulty in breathing, noisy respirations, extremely shallow respirations, may indicate need for tracheostomy and assisted respirations.

Oxygen should not be given routinely as it may mask severe respiratory insufficiency. When it is ordered the need for its continuance should be checked hourly.

Secretions. Record amount and type. Atropine is never used as it makes secretions tenacious and viscous and predisposes to bronchial obstruction and atelectasis. Furthermore, excessive bronchial fluid is more likely to be oedema fluid than true bronchial secretion and atropine does not affect excretion of oedema fluid.

Suction should be performed with pre-sterilized catheters of small gauge. Whistle-tip type is better than one with lateral holes. Method of use is important — catheter inserted while pinched closed and then withdrawn unpinched and with a rotary movement. It should not be jabbed back and forth. Catheter enters right bronchus readily. To enter left bronchus patient may be placed on left side or head turned to the right. Instillation of sodium bicarbonate should not be done as it paralyses ciliary movement.

Mouth. Frequent washouts with swabs on forceps and a mild antiseptic. Swabs should be squeezed moderately dry. Denture plates should always be removed. Peppermint cream or petroleum jelly applied to lips.

Eyes. Often partly open and need careful protection from abrasion. Make sure bedclothes etc. cannot rub cornea. Instil castor oil drop twice daily alternating with antibiotic eye drop twice daily. Light pad bandaged over eyes may be necessary.

Skin. Keep clean and well dried. Depend on frequent turning to prevent pressure sores. Avoid soapy massaging and methylated spirit rubs which dry the skin too much.

Bladder. Retention or incontinence is common. Occasionally automatic emptying of bladder occurs every two hours and a urinal in position at the appropriate time can save much anxiety

(urinals should not be left permanently in position). If catheriza-
tion is performed every aseptic precaution must be taken. Catheter should be connected immediately to underwater seal containing formalin 40 per cent. Catheter should be clamped and clamp
released every two hours. Bladder should be emptied completely
on each occasion by manual compression of suprapubic area.
Meatal toilets performed twice daily with chlorhexidine.
Changes of catheter are avoided. Polythene is less irritant than
rubber. Small size catheter better than large. Danger of urinary
infection high unless great care taken.

Urine. Careful record of amount passed. Doctor informed if it
falls below 100 ml per hour. Tested daily for albumin and
acetone. Micro-examination for organisms and pus cells.

Fluids. Hydration maintained, preferably by intragastric tube
as the variety and quantity is much more flexible than by
intravenous route. Stomach aspirated two hourly immediately
prior to feeding. Equivalent amount to aspirate taken into
account when estimating needs. If aspirant is small it may be
returned with the feed.

Physiotherapy. Limbs put through fall range of movement
three times daily. Chest percussed to dislodge mucus. Suction
applied immediately after.

Observations and charts. Temperature, pulse, respirations,
blood pressure, fluid intake and output, pupil reaction and size,
state of muscle tone. *Changes* in any of these are significant.

9. Collagen Diseases

Definition. Group of diseases affecting many systems simultaneously. All have immunological changes affecting connective tissues. Often difficult to delineate sharply between them. Inflammatory reactions occur wherever connective tissues found, i.e. in all organs to a variable extent. Disease often chronic, relapsing, progressive and crippling. Diagnostic features rarely specific. Immunofluorescent techniques revealing more information about them. As research progresses into immune reactions, immunoglobulins, complement, knowledge of collagen diseases broadens.

Rheumatoid arthritis

Systemic disease in which inflammation of joints is prominent symptom.

Cause. Unknown. Auto-immunity being investigated as cause. Familial tendency. More common in temperate climates where cold and damp occur. Women more affected than men (3:1). No age immune but diagnosis usually after 40 years of age.

Pathology. Inflammatory oedema, excessive capillarity, followed by granulations, necrosis and fibrosis of synovial membranes. Granulations invade hyaline cartilage. Fibrinous bridges develop between articular surfaces. These may ossify later. Similar changes may occur in tendon sheaths, bursae, subcutaneous nodules, pericardium, heart valves.

Signs and symptoms. Early — rapid onset of fatigue, anorexia, weight loss. Transient aches and pains in muscles and joints.

Later — joints painful, red, swollen and stiff. Hands, knees and ankles commonly affected first. Unnatural bending of joints follows tendon shortening and prolonged muscle spasm. Aching and stiffness of muscles common after rest or inactivity. Skin of extremities cold, pale and sweaty. Nodules in skin occur in 10–20 per cent of cases — rounded, painless lumps which are mobile and occur over or near pressure areas and near joints. Moderate anaemia common. ESR raised during active disease. Raised temperature accompanies acute phases.

Diagnosis. Presence of rheumatoid factor in gamma globulin is suggestive. X-ray examination shows osteoporosis, narrowing of joint spaces, erosion of hyaline cartilage.

Treatment. Psychological factors important. Patient warned that treatment must be prolonged but encouraged to take an optimistic attitude. Best results when treatment started early.

Rest. Complete bed rest while pain severe and temperature elevated. In less severe cases, moderate exercise encouraged. Patient should have 8–10 hours sleep a night.

Physiotherapy. Exercises designed to prevent joint stiffness and delay ankylosis as long as possible, to prevent deformities and to maintain or increase muscle power.

While confined to bed all joints put through full range of movements. 'Muscle setting' exercises for quadriceps and gluteals to prevent muscle wasting. Bed should be firm, without sag. Patient should sleep flat with one small pillow. Local heat prior to exercises reduces pain and muscle spasm. Exercises of hands and feet may be performed while parts immersed in wax bath. Limbs may be splinted during sleep to prevent deformity. Exercises may be continued for years. Patient must be taught need for regular performance at home with visits to physiotherapy department for checking progress and early detection of deformity. Constant encouragement necessary.

Pain. Primary aim is to treat inflammatory cause of pain rather than mere suppression with analgesics. Salicylates, phenylbutazone, indomethacin, ibuprofen and corticosteroids, are used. Aspirin given as a course of therapy and not merely when pain becomes severe. 2–3 g daily in divided doses. Gastric irritation avoided by giving soluble aspirin at mealtimes. Phenylbutazone (Butazolidine) 300–400 mg daily. Discontinued after 7 days if pain not relieved as dangers of drug are serious — agranulocytosis, anaemia, thrombocytopenia, peptic ulcer, salt retention, skin rashes. Indomethacin (Indocid) 25 mg q.i.d.

Corticosteroids. Much controversy over their use. Often dramatic improvement of symptoms but disease process is not halted and possible complications severe — peptic ulceration, osteoporosis, rapid spread of infections. Prednisone commonly used, 10–15 mg daily. Dose kept to minimum with gradual reduction every 6 months to see if spontaneous remission of symptoms had occurred. Occasionally, injection into joint cavity is beneficial causing relief from pain and stiffness for about 10 days.

Gold salts. These may give relief but are not curative. Regime — dosage increased weekly 10 mg, 25 mg, 50 mg, and then 50 mg weekly until a total of 1 g gold salt has been given. Reactions are common — skin eruptions, suppression of red marrow activity, nephritis. Blood examined monthly. Urine examined before each injection.

Still's disease

Condition closely resembling rheumatoid arthritis but occurs in children 5–10 years.

Cause. Unknown. May be auto-immune disease.

Signs and symptoms. Similar onset to rheumatoid arthritis in adults but knees and wrists affected initially rather than fingers. Nodules absent. Lymph nodes, spleen and liver enlarged. Temperature raised. Remittent type of fever. Leucocytosis.

Treatment. As for rheumatoid arthritis. (Salicylates do not relieve pain).

Polymyalgia rheumatica

Weakness, stiffness, muscle tenderness affecting proximal muscle of shoulder girdle more than pelvic.

Cause. Unknown.

Signs and symptoms. Most common in middle aged women. Onset usually abrupt with pain, aching, tenderness over larger muscle bulks. Joints not affected though patient wrongly localised the stiffness at joints. Stiffness worst on waking. May need help to get out of bed and dress. Pain, and stiffness lessen throughout day. Improved by massage and warmth. May be fever and weight loss.

Pathological tests almost always show a high erythrocyte sedimentation rate with few other abnormalities.

Diagnosis. Indicated by physical findings, lack of positive pathology and presence of rapid ESR. Often association with giant cell arteritis.

Treatment. Rapid and dramatic improvement on low dose corticosteroids, prednisolone 10–15 mg daily. May need to continue for months. Maintenance dose discovered by reducing to least amount daily which prevents relapse. Readjusted every three months. May be possible to stop steroid for long periods. Duration of treatment often depends on duration of disease prior to diagnosis. If giant cell arteritis suspected biopsy of temporal artery performed for confirmation and much higher doses of prednisolone used to prevent blindness.

Polymyositis (Dermatomyositis)

Condition in which skin and voluntary muscle undergo inflammatory change. High incidence of subsequent malignant occurence.

Cause. Unknown. Lymphocytes sensitised to muscle cells.

Signs and symptoms. Usually insidious onset with muscular aching, weakness, slight temperature, erythematous patches on extensor surfaces which may desquamate and later become hard and indurated. Mild anaemia, rapid ESR, raised SGOT, CPK and aldolase.

Muscle weakness usually general but specific muscles cause special problems, e.g. diaphragm resulting in respiratory insufficiency; extrinsic muscles of eyes causing diplopia, failure to accommodate; pharyngeal muscles causing difficulty in swallowing, inhalation of food and asphyxia.

Diagnosis. Electromyography and muscle biopsy.

Treatment. Supportive only. Corticosteroids, e.g. prednisolone up to 60 mg daily until CPK normal, then maintenance dose. Tracheostomy and assisted respiration may be required.

Prognosis. Usually slowly crippling but may run fulminating fatal course especially in children.

Systemic lupus erythematosus (SLE)

Inflammatory changes in connective tissues throughout body.
Cause. Unknown. Multiple auto-antibodies found. To red cell

protein, platelets, thrombin, nuclear material. Also often high titres to various viruses, e.g. of glandular fever, measles, influenza, hepatitis. Hereditary predisposition likely. Condition occurs in both identical twins, anti-nuclear factor found in other relatives.

Signs and symptoms. All systems affected to some degree. General weakness, weight loss, fatigue. Rash, classically symmetrically distributed over nose and cheeks — butterfly distribution. More marked wherever skin exposed to sunlight. Splenomegaly in 25 per cent. Pleurisy and atelectasis, pericarditis, myocarditis, ulceration of any or all mucous surfaces, interference with digestive function, malabsorption.

Proteinuria may herald lupus nephritis which can go on to nephrotic syndrome and renal failure. Nervous system involvement may cause convulsions, hemiplegia or psychoses.

Diagnosis. Often delayed because of multiple symptomology. Suggestive findings are rapid ESR, positive Coombs test, raised serum globulin with lymphopenia, and reduced levels of complement. Antinuclear factor present in 97 per cent. Finding of LE cells in special preparations confirms diagnosis but their absence does not deny it.

Treatment. Generally unsatisfactory. Corticosteroids help to ameliorate symptoms but do not cure. In early stages 10–15 mg prednisolone daily may be enough. When vital organs affected — heart, CNS, kidneys — high dosage given — 60–70 mg daily until improvement allows gradual reduction.

Cytotoxic drugs used with caution. Long term use of these may cause side effects worse than SLE.

Prognosis. Generally poor. Episodic pattern with gradually worsening residual ability. Occasionally rapid, fulminating course.

Periarteritis nodosa

Progressive weakening of medium sized arteries with necrosis, fibrotic change, and aneurysm formation. Widespread organ involvement — kidneys, lungs, heart, skin, intestines, muscles, nerves, with multiple symptoms.

Cause. Unknown. Immunological development to many antigens found — viruses, tissue cells, some drugs.

Signs and symptoms. Often hypertension earliest sign with renal insufficiency, variety of muscular aches, pains, stiffness and weakness, malaise, weight loss. Asthma may arise suddenly, as may congestive cardiac failure, and unusual skin eruptions.

Laboratory findings include raised ESR, leukocytosis, anaemia, raised serum globulin level. Urine usually shows blood cells, albumen, pus cells, casts.

Diagnosis. Not easy. Biopsy may show necrotic arterioles. Anteriography may show multiple aneurysms.

Treatment. Prednisolone. High dosage initially reducing to maintenance doses.

Prognosis. Often rapidly fatal. May be slowly progressive.

Scleraderma

Gradual increase in collagen fibres in skin, mucous membranes and many internal organs.

Cause. Unknown. Anti-nuclear factor commonly present.

Signs and symptoms. Gradual thickening of skin which becomes stiff, inelastic. May be preceded years before by Raynaud's phenomenon and excessive sweating. Ulceration of fingers and toes, infection, pigmentation. Oesophageal involvement causes dysphagia, gastro-oesophageal reflux, heart burn. Thickening of intestinal walls, causes difficulty in peristalsis, malabsorption, constipation, pulmonary fibrosis reduces lung compliance. Respiratory infection and failure may be cause of death. Myocardial involvement leads to arrhythmias and congestive cardiac failure. Renal involvement is revealed by albuminuria and renal failure.

Diagnosis. No certain diagnostic tests. X-ray shows calcification in skin, osteoporosis, phalangeal destruction. Auto-antibodies present in most cases.

Treatment. Nil specific. Corticosteroids if muscles involved. Vasodilators may be helpful in Raynaud's disease.

Prognosis. Usually slowly progressive.

Reiter's syndrome

Combination of urethritis, arthritis, conjunctivitis, and various mucocutaneous lesions.

Cause. Unknown. Possibly viral.

Signs and symptoms. Commonly arises in young men with history of recent sexual intercourse. Urethritis caused dysuria without urethral discharge. Arthritis usually of large joints. May persist long after all other symptoms disappear. Skin lesions variable. May resemble psoriasis.

Diagnosis. No specific test but often HLA antigen 27 present.

Treatment. Symptomatic. Anti-inflammatory drugs effective in relieving arthritic pain — aspirin, phenylbutazone, indomethacin.

Prognosis. Spontaneous cure common. Relapse occur. Occasionally joint involvement progresses to ankylosing spondylitis.

Index

Cor pulmonale, 14
Corticosteroids in ulcerative colitis, 93
Coumadin, 46
Cretinism, 138
Crohn's disease, 88
Cross matching, 46
Croup, 51
Cushing's syndrome, 136, 155
Cycloserine, 63
Cystitis, 125
Cystostocopy, 108
Cytotoxic agents, 40, 42

Deep X-rays in hyperthyroidism, 141
Degenerative joint disease, 166
De-Nol, 81
Deposits in urine, 110
Dermatomyositis, 195
Diabetic coma, 151
Diabetes, complications in, 151
Diabetes, insipidus, 136
Diabetic ketosis, 151
Diabetes mellitus, 145
Diabetic societies, 150
Diabetes, stabilization, 146
Diabenese, 148
Dialysis, peritoneal, 113
Diazoxide, 24
Dibenzyline, 159
Dicoumarol, 46
Dialysis, 112
Diazoxide, 21
Diet in diabetes, 149
Digitalis, 6
Digitalis, as diuretic, 132
Digitalis in A.F., 2
Dilantin, 183
Dindevan, 46
Diphenylhydantoin, 183
Disopyramide, 3, 8
Disseminated sclerosis, 184
Diuretics, modes of action, 130
Diuretics in nephrotic syndrome, 116
Diverticulitis, 94
Diverticulum of bladder, 125
Diverticulum, Meckel's, 92

Donor, universal, 46
Double kidney, 122
Double ureter, 123
Dramamine, 186
Drug stomatitis, 74
Dumping syndrome, 86
Duodenoscopy, 80
Duogastrone, 81
Dwarfism, 134
Dymerhydrinate, 186
Dysentery, 86
Dyspepsia, 78

Early morning specimen of urine, 111
ECG, see Electrocardiogram,
  in heart block, 4
  in myocardial infarction, 16
  in atrial fibrillation, 2
Ectopic bladder, 123
Ectopic kidney, 122
Edecril, 131
Education in diabetes, 149
Eisenmenger's syndrome, 26
Electrocardiogram, 1
Embolism, 14
Embolism, pulmonary, 58
Emphysema, 57
Empyema, 66
Endocarditis — acute bacterial, 10
  subacute bacterial, 10
Endocrine system, 133
Enuresis, nocturnal, 123
Enzymes, in liver disease, 96
  in myocardial infarction, 16
Epididymitis, 129
Epilepsy, 182
  stages, 183
Epispadias, 127
Erythroblastosis fetalis, 34, 48
Ethacrynic acid, 131
Ethambutol, 63
Ethylnoradrenaline, 55
Eumydrine, 85

Facial paralysis, 187
Factor VIII deficiency, 44
Fallot's tetralogy, 26
Ferrivenin, 36